ETHICS

ASPECTS OF NURSING CARE

ETHICS

ASPECTS OF
NURSING CARE

Edited by

Verena Tschudin BSc (Hons), RGN, RM,
Dip. Counselling

Illustrations by Richard Smith

Scutari Press · London

First published 1993

British Library Cataloguing in Publication Data
Aspects of Nursing Care
  I. Tschudin, Verena
  174
  ISBN 1–871364–79–5

Contents

Acknowledgements

The publisher and editor wish to thank the Voluntary Euthanasia Society for permission to reproduce the Advance Directive and the Royal College of Nursing for permission to reproduce Living Wills — Guidance for Nurses, both of which appear in chapter four.

Contributors

June Andrews RMN, RGN, MA(Glas), MA(Nottm)

Assistant Director, Policy and Research, Royal College of Nursing

Paul Cain MA

Lecturer, University of Reading

Davina Gilbert RGN

Renal Unit, Hammersmith Hospital

Jennifer Iliffe CQSW

Senior Practitioner Social Worker, Royal Brompton National Heart and Lung Hospital

Pamela Swan RGN, Dip.N, BA

Clinical Nurse Specialist, Royal Brompton National Heart and Lung Hospital

Preface

Ethics is not only at the heart of nursing, it *is* the heart of nursing. Ethics is about what is right and good. Nursing and caring are synonymous, and the way in which care is carried out is ethically decisive. How a patient is addressed, cared for and treated must be right not only by ordinary standards of care, but also by ethical principles.

These ethical principles have not always been addressed clearly, but now patients, nurses, doctors and all types of health care personnel are questioning their care in the light of ethics. Their starting points and approaches are different, but their 'results' are remarkably similar. The individual person matters and the care given and received has to be human and humanising.

The way in which the contributors to this volume, and others in the series, address their subject is also individual and unique. Their brief was simply that what they wrote should be applicable to practising nurses. Each chapter reflects the personal style and approach of the writer. This is what gives this series its distinctive character and strength, and provides the reader with the opportunity to see different approaches working. It is hoped that this will encourage readers to think that their own way of understanding ethics and behaving ethically is also acceptable and worthwhile. Theories and principles are important, and so are their interpretation and application. That is a job for everybody, not just the experts: experts can point the way – as in this series of books – but all nurses need to be challenged and encouraged.

Emphasis is laid in all the chapters on the individual nurse and patient or client. Ethics 'happens' between and among people, and, by the authors bringing their own experience to bear on their chapters, they show how ethics works in relationships.

Great achievements often start with a small idea quite different from the end result, and so it is with this series of books. The initial proposal is almost unrecognisable in the final product. Many people contributed to the growth of the idea, many more were involved in implementing it, and I hope that even more will benefit from it.

My particular thanks go to Geoff Hunt, Director of the National Centre for Nursing and Midwifery Ethics, for his advice and help with this series.

Verena Tschudin

CHAPTER 1

Abortion and Contraception

June Andrews

Abortion and contraception must have been practised since time immemorial. History relates more of the failures than the successes of various practices. Life and death are so completely tied up in the subject that the issues have rarely been easy to describe or defend.

An understanding of biology, traditions and the law helps us to understand the subject more objectively. The ethical implications are described in this chapter from the point of view of different people, based on case histories. This allows various aspects to come to light which may otherwise be hidden in often one-sided arguments. Some rhetorical questions in the last part of the chapter invite readers to answer their own thoughts on this topic.

Abortion and contraception are ready subjects for ethical debate. People have very strong views about sex, death, religion, law and politics. The arguments seem very new and related to modern technology: the contraceptive pill, AIDS, the use of fetal material for experimentation and infertility treatment are all relatively recent phenomena and the law has responded to them. Nurses are faced with new and complicated situations every day. Nevertheless we must remember that ever since the time when humans realised the connection between sexual intercourse and pregnancy, women (and some men) have addressed the issue of how to interrupt the process and avoid the birth of a child.

In order to have a sensible discussion about what is

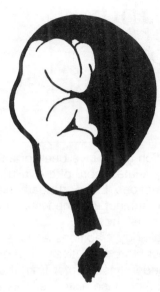

involved, it is very important to agree on what is being said. Emotive language can muddy the water and prevent us from seeing what we are saying. The technical terms that are used can be misinterpreted or used in different ways by different authors. So when you begin to think about abortion and contraception, it is important to know the basic biological details and agree what words you will use. You will be able to tell a great deal about what people feel from the language that they use about the subject.

It is also helpful to know what the legal position is. That something is legal and permissible under the law does not make it ethical. The law is a strange mixture of rules that are apparently written on tablets of stone in statute, rules that can be inferred from what judges have said, and rules that we work to but which have never been tested. Examples of all of these can be cited in relation to abortion. The reasons why the law stands as it is are also of interest because the intentions of the law makers may not always seem to be reflected in the final law.

In order to understand the legal position, it is important to know some of the history of the ideas involved, so you need to know a little about the cultural and religious beliefs of the people who made the laws and the people who are subject to them. You must be aware of the personal beliefs that you bring to the discussion, and understand why it is you feel the way you do. Once you have an understanding of what the issues are and what your own position is, you can look at examples of practical ethical problems in nursing people who are undergoing abortion and choosing contraception, and you will be able to identify and understand the views of others.

In this chapter we will follow this route, looking at the biology, the law and the history before looking at some real ethical dilemmas.

Biology

The **ovum** (egg) and **sperm** are produced by the ovary and the testis respectively. The ovum and sperm, or **gametes**, divide and reduce their chromosome content by half. This process makes gametes unique among cells. At conception the sperm passes through the egg wall and the chromosomes of the sperm and ovum then join together. The fertilised egg is called the **zygote**. It divides into many cells and by the fourth day grows into a **morula**. When the morula develops a cavity and starts to implant into the wall of the uterus, it is called a **blastocyst**. The outer part of the blastocyst becomes the placenta and fetal membranes. Inner cells become the **embryo**. The whole of the product of conception can be called the **conceptus**.

The conceptus is referred to as the **pre-embryo** for the first two weeks. After the eighth week it is called a **fetus**.

Around the fourteenth day after fertilisation the **primitive streak** is formed on the embryo, and the three basic elements which will form tissue can be identified. The **neural plate** is identified on the twenty-sixth day. The heart starts to beat on the twenty-second day. By the seventh week the embryo looks human, with distinct fingers and toes. The gender of the fetus can be distinguished by ultrasound scan at 12 weeks after fertilisation.

It appears that the fetus is able to feel some pain at 14–18 weeks. Movements can be felt by the mother at 16–20 weeks and this is known as **quickening**. There is much discussion about when a fetus is likely to be viable as an infant. Infants born prematurely can be kept alive after 24 weeks in the womb, and accepted good practice for termination of pregnancy has been to act before then, but 24 weeks is now a significant time in abortion law.

Some women who are in tune with their bodies, or who have been taking their temperature regularly, are aware of the changes which take place when the egg is released from the ovary. A slight pain known as **mittelschmertz** is often experienced at that time, as is a change in temperature. Some women become aware very quickly when an egg has been fertilised, and are conscious of the bodily changes that occur as hormone levels shift and the body starts to adapt to the new challenge, even before they have missed a menstrual period. Sometimes a woman experiences her entire pregnancy without becoming aware of it. She may have another plausible reason for any weight gain or the absence of a period of menstruation (such as the menopause), and comes to the doctor with abdominal pain and in labour. Social pressures may cause some women to deny the fact of pregnancy and hide it as long as possible. These and other factors influence the form of contraception that a woman will choose, and will influence whether and when she will request an abortion.

Methods of Birth Control

Between sexual intercourse (and I use that general term because it can happen in a number of ways) and the birth of a child there are many points at which the process can be interrupted:

- *Ovulation* — can be prevented by hormone pills or sterilisation (mechanical).
- *Abstinence.*
- *Intercourse* — mechanical barrier (cap or condom), withdrawal before ejaculation, timing (to avoid ovulation time), sterilisation (male vasectomy).
- *After intercourse* — morning–after hormonal pill.
- *After fertilisation* — intra-uterine contraceptive device, IUCD, (to prevent implantation).
- *After implantation* — menstrual aspiration, vacuum aspiration, prostaglandin or induced abortion, dilation and evacuation, hysterectomy (eg if uterine cancer is discovered or sterilisation is taking place).
- *During birth* — the fetus may be deliberately destroyed or the infant neglected.

Abortion is in itself illegal in the UK, so if any of these procedures can be described as abortion, it can only be done if it is one of the exceptional cases covered by the *Abortion Act* 1986 and Amendments. Killing a child is also illegal (*Infant Life [Preservation] Act* 1929), so if any of these can be interpreted as killing a viable child, that is illegal too. Contraception is unacceptable to some people on religious and moral grounds so anything in the above list (apart from abstinence) may be off limits for some people.

Interruption of the process can take place at any time before the gametes fuse, between fertilisation and implantation, after implantation and before the organs form, or between the formation of some rudimentary organs and the development of a creature that could (with some basic help) survive outside the womb. It may be the case that the fetus has reached the stage of development at which it could survive, but it would have to be killed unless the mother was prepared to die in getting it into the world.

Religious Traditions of Abortion and Contraception

In ancient Egypt women are supposed to have inserted mud as a mechanical barrier to prevent sperm reaching the cervix during intercourse. The Bible describes the practice of seed being 'spilled on the ground', that is ejaculation outside the vagina. The men who interpreted God's will for early Christians accepted the view that the Old Testament law forbids abortion. Prevention of birth was the same as murder. Killing someone who was about to be a person was the same as killing a person. Scholars now say that this idea was derived erroneously from purification rites described in the book of Leviticus.

The problem for the ancient Christians was working out how to get to heaven (Dunstan and Sellar 1988). If being baptised was essential, it meant that the unbaptised would go to hell, which seemed a cruel fate for the unbaptised unborn child. It would be a sin for any woman, and for the abortionist if she had help in procuring the abortion, to cause the loss of a soul. St Augustine taught that the unbaptised fetus was lost, but Thomas Aquinas said that when quickening was observed the soul had entered the fetus and until that time there was no soul to be saved. Thus a distinction was made between the fetus *formatus* and the fetus *informatus*. The fetus became formatus when movement was observed either by the mother or by external observers. If the fetus was destroyed at this late time, its soul would be lost. In

Roman law a distinction was made between early and late abortion. In 1148 Canon Law, the law of the Church, came into line with Roman Law and the differentiation of formatus and informatus was codified. The destruction of the fetus *formatus* was a serious crime.

In modern times Roman Catholics have been required to behave as if the soul enters the pre-embryo at the time of fertilisation. Abstinence and timing of intercourse to avoid fertilisation are acceptable, although this was not always the case. Abortion before the time of quickening was once not regarded as an unforgivable sin, but a statement by Pope Pius IX, and the declaration of the infallibility of the Pope at the First Vatican Council in 1869, made the ruling more stringent. The 1968 encyclical *Humanae Vitae* sent out the clear message to the faithful that birth control is a sin. Some priests, especially those working in areas of the world where there is great poverty, express views opposing this. Other religions have objections to birth control which range from a feeling that its existence would encourage fornication to a belief that taking any life at all is wrong.

The moral tradition of the Church 'attempted to grade the protection accorded to the nascent human being depending on the stages of its development' (Dunstan and Sellar 1988):

- *Christian* — killing is a capital offence because human beings are made in the image of God (Genesis 9:6)
  - (i) Roman Catholic — since 1986 abortion has been condemned.
    Ectopic pregnancies are dealt with by 'double effect'*. The doctrine of original sin** is upheld.
  - (ii) Protestant — there is considerable variation in the attitude to abortion, and there is discussion as to whether an embryo has personal rights.

(iii) Orthodox — views similar to the Roman Catholic that killing the fetus is the same as murder.

- Jewish — the unborn child has a right to life in different stages from the moment of conception, to be set aside only in exceptional circumstances, such as serious hazard to the mother.
- Islamic — Islamic writing suggests that the unformed fetus (before 120 days) is not yet a human being.
- Hindu — Hindu scripts specifically mention abortion as a serious crime. Ancient writings make an exception when the life of the mother is at risk.

* Double effect. This is used to justify doing something that would normally be wrong, by claiming that it is being done for an innocent reason. The removal of the fallopian tube which will terminate an ectopic pregnancy is done because the tube is diseased and not in order to sacrifice the fetus in the interest of the mother.

** Doctrine of original sin. This is the teaching that every person inherits the sin of Adam and Eve and will be damned if not baptised.

The law in the United Kingdom largely reflects the beliefs of the Christian church, although our society is enriched by a large number of cultures and religions. A rule against taking life is common to most religious systems of belief, and the interesting differences come in the area where religions will allow exceptions to be made. These exceptions are often rationalised according to the apparent reason behind the rule. If taking life is always wrong, any abortion is wrong. If killing potential persons because of their value as individuals is wrong, pre-conceptual birth control may be acceptable. If the purpose of marriage is to produce children, birth control within marriage (or recreational as opposed to procreational sexual intercourse) is wrong. The interpretation of the Biblical exhortation to 'be fruitful and multiply' (Genesis 1:28; 9:1) is that anything other than active procreation within marriage is sinful, ruling out certain sexual practices, or contraception and abortion.

History of Abortion Laws in the United Kingdom

Prior to 1803, abortion before quickening was not against the law in England. The methods used were crude and dangerous, and often involved the woman poisoning herself with lead or mechanically damaging her internal organs with a contaminated foreign object, then dying of the subsequent infection. In 1803 it became a criminal offence to cause an abortion at any stage, punishable by flogging, life imprisonment or death. The death penalty was dropped in 1838. In 1861 a major piece of legislation was produced, *The Offences Against the Person Act*, which assumed that abortion is always a criminal and immoral act. It has been suggested that up until then the purpose of the law in this area was to protect women against harm, but the new Act seemed to focus on the sanctity of life of the fetus.

The Infant Life (Preservation) Act 1929 allowed the fetus to be destroyed 'in good faith with the intention of saving the life of the mother'. This Act was not changed by the *Abortion Act* introduced to Parliament in 1967. In 1961, before the *Abortion Act* and 100 years after the *Offences Against The Person Act*, 2300 abortions took place within the NHS in that one year, performed by doctors in the interest of the health of the mother. This could include consideration of her mental health, following a ruling in 1938. (A doctor performed an abortion on a 14–year–old survivor of multiple rape, at the request of her father, and was acquitted at trial [R v Bourne 1938.]) So why did women and their doctors need the *Abortion Act*? The avail-

ability of abortions was limited and women with few
resources were still dying from dangerous self-induced or
'back street' abortions. Criminals were making a lot of
money out of dangerous procedures that could have been
done safely by a doctor in a clinic. A woman with money
could pay for a doctor to do it secretly if the doctor was
prepared to risk the legal penalties in order to help her,
but many poorer women died.

It is interesting to look at some of the debates that took
place around the Act in the 1960s. Some of the supporters
felt that legislation would make the situation more equitable, but others, who were more conservative, felt that
it was needed to control the size of families and to stop
irresponsible women from carelessly reproducing. In the
debate in support of abortion Lord Silkin described categories of women who might benefit from it, including
women with epilepsy, shop lifters, women whose hus-
bands were drunkards or in prison and others who were
'not a fit person to be in charge of children'.

There have been further changes in the law since the
Act. The *Abortion Regulations* 1991 came into effect on
April 1st 1991. The *Human Fertilisation and Embryology Act*
1990 amended the 1967 *Abortion Act* by reducing the time
limit for abortions to 24 weeks from 28 weeks, in line
with good practice. In line with actual practice, it allows
for termination at any stage in the case of danger to the
mother or possible abnormality of the child. It allows the
destruction of some of the fetuses in a multiple pregnancy,
and the use of abortifacient drugs in places that are not
licensed for abortion. It also removes the anomaly of the
28 week presumption of fetal viability in the *Infant Life
(Preservation) Act* 1929 (which never applied in Scotland).

Because of the wording of the 1967 Act there was
anxiety among nurses about their legal position when
assisting with abortion procedures. The DHSS produced
guidelines for the procedure, but it was felt that nurses

might be accused of 'procuring miscarriage'. The case RCN v DHSS (1981) gave nurses a defence under the *Offences Against the Person Act* 1861. The RCN had felt that nurses taking part in the proceedings were not protected by the law to do what the DHSS was asking of them and they might be prosecuted. RCN v DHSS established that nurses were able to work within the *Abortion Act* without breaking the other law.

The Conscience Clause

A substantial number of health care professionals have religious or other personal objections to abortion, and legislation within this area reflects this. The conscience clause (Section 4 of the *Abortion Act*) provides that 'no person shall be under any duty, whether by contract, by statutory or other legal requirement to participate in any treatment authorised by this Act to which he has a conscientious objection, provided that in any legal proceeding the burden of proof of conscience shall rest upon the person claiming it.' The conscience clause does not relieve a person of 'any duty to participate in any treatment which is necessary to save the life or to prevent grave permanent injury to the physical or mental health of a pregnant woman'.

Nurses have the protection of the *Abortion Act* when they accept delegated instructions from a registered medical practitioner and carry out the treatment in accordance with his or her directions. The medical practitioner remains in overall charge of the case throughout.

The protection of the clause is only given to those nurses who 'participate in any treatment'. In one case the clause was tested by a secretary who refused to write a letter referring a patient to a consultant about a possible termination. Both the Court of Appeal and the House of

Lords accepted the health authority's argument that the
words 'participating in treatment' referred to 'actually
taking part in treatment administered in a hospital or
other approved place . . . for the purposes of terminating
pregnancies'. So even if she did not like it, the secretary
had to write the letter (Janaway v Salford Health Authority 1988).

Practical Ethics

Abortion is a violent act. On both sides of the debate
about its morality there are powerful feelings. Before
reading the case in point below, you might remember this
advice taken from the start of Richard Rowson's book *An
Introduction to Ethics for Nurses* (1990):

> Understand a view before judging it. First make sure you
> understand the view then think about whether or not you
> agree with it.

In reading the story below of a pregnant woman, her
boyfriend, her husband and her health carers, you may
have a strong view about what they ought to do. After
describing the situation I will speculate about what some
of the people involved are thinking and feeling and why.
At the end I will present an analysis of some of the points
of view that give rise to these feelings and beliefs.

- Agnes Barnes was a 38-year-old married nurse specialist
  who decided that she longed to have a daughter so would
  try to have a child before it was too late. She and her
  husband had always used contraception and she had used
  the IUCD for the last year. She had her coil removed and
  started to take her temperature regularly. During this time
  she was going through a lot of changes at work and in her
  personal feelings, and she thought that was why when she
  met an old boyfriend, Colin, on a weekend trip to a class

reunion, she went to bed with him. She discovered that she was pregnant, but decided to assume that it was nothing to do with her fling with Colin.

Because of her age she went through a planned programme of screening for malformation, chorion villus biopsy, amniocentesis, blood sampling and anomaly scanning at 18–20 weeks. She had a good service from the hospital but unavoidable delays meant that it was 28 weeks before she discovered that her doctor suspected that the fetus was male and abnormal. She was told that he would probably always be very dependent and might not live beyond 13 years. In her distress she went to talk to Colin and was made to feel worse when she discovered that he was a member of a pro-life organisation. That was why he had not used contraception. Colin felt sure that the child was his and he demanded that she should have it.

Her husband David, who was a nurse for people with learning difficulties, decided that if the child was handicapped he would give up work to be a house husband and care for him. Agnes told him nothing about Colin but insisted that she wanted a termination. David, who had already felt the fetus kicking against his hand when he held Agnes close to him, was shocked. He had already started to think of the fetus as Edward. Agnes was sick of the whole mess. Apart from anything else her pregnancy was making her feel ill and she was under pressure at work because of the amount of time she was having to take off to attend clinics. She just wished that it was all over.

Do you think that Agnes should have an abortion? A woman is not actually in a position to choose to have an abortion. The decision always rests with two doctors, but of course the doctors would listen very carefully to what she wanted. On the face of it, she would be a candidate for a termination of pregnancy under the *Abortion Act* 1967. The doctor could show that her condition was such that having the child would harm her health and that there

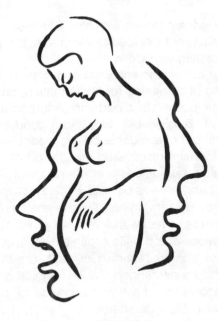

was a grave danger of the child being handicapped. Best practice usually demands that the decision be made before 24 weeks, but if the danger to the mother is sufficiently grave, the decision can be made after that. The dilemma for the doctor is twofold. Firstly, the nature of the disability that the potential child has must be so great that its life would not be worth living. Although it is the case that virtually any child is viable to a certain extent, and no-one would relish the prospect of a short and painful existence for a severely handicapped child, there are many people with severe learning disabilities or physical disabilities whose life is of value to both themselves and their families and society. Although doctors are allowed to take the disability into consideration, they still have to consider whether it is a *serious* enough consideration. Secondly, the doctor has to decide whether or not Agnes's health is likely to suffer. It has been suggested that carers do suffer significantly more from depression, anxiety and the physical symptoms that go along with those conditions. One might also say that the situation is so stressful for Agnes that her mental health will suffer, and the doctor is able to take this into consideration too. But could it be argued that because Agnes has got resources and skills, a supportive husband (and even the support of a boyfriend if that fails), her fear of mental distress at the birth of the baby is an exaggerated one? Could it also be argued that the birth of the child is in fact mainly an inconvenience to Agnes, who has only ever expressed an interest in having a female child?

Do you think Agnes would be more interested in carrying the fetus to term and then giving birth to a child if it were a girl? If Agnes confessed to that, might it paradoxically make the doctor less inclined to terminate her boy? Termination for reasons solely related to a preferred gender would be illegal.

Colin, her friend, might try to argue with Agnes that she is taking a very serious step by killing this fetus. A unique person has been created by the fusion of (somebody's) individual gametes and she would have the loss of that person on her conscience for ever. Agnes might reply that this would not be the first 'potential person' that she has destroyed because she has been wearing an IUCD for the last year and to her knowledge could have been pregnant every month during that year and disposed of the pre-embryo by stopping it embedding itself in her uterus. By disposing of this fetus she is being totally consistent.

Colin might feel that he should be in a position to prevent Agnes legally from having a termination, out of some sense that perhaps the child is his property as well. There is no legal precedent for a father preventing the termination taking place (C v S 1988). Even supposing that Colin could at this stage prove his paternity, he would be unable to act in the interest of keeping the fetus alive.

He could do his best to persuade Agnes to continue with the pregnancy, by offering her support, by suggesting that the child should be adopted at birth, or by pointing out that there may be a danger of difficulty with subsequent pregnancies and therefore her best chance of having the much desired female child is to continue with this pregnancy. He might argue that rather than there being a danger to her health if she has the child, there is more danger to her health if she does not have the child because of the risk of depression and anxiety later.

Apart from the fact that he is in ignorance about the affair, David, the husband, is in a disadvantaged position. He cannot do anything in law to stop the termination of pregnancy. His wife will have no difficulty persuading a doctor that she should have one. He knows that the justification for decriminalising abortion in 1967 was that it was supposed to benefit mothers of large families, women carrying handicapped children and those whose health was endangered by pregnancy. He also knows that in fact the typical woman seeking an abortion today is young, single, with no previous children and carrying a healthy baby. Given his wife's age and what he perceives as the prejudice in society against disabled people, he knows that it is a difficult position. He also knows that following the Arthur case in 1981, even if the child is born, its life is not yet safe. In that case, a baby with Down's Syndrome was given sedating drugs and died within 63 hours of birth. The doctor was charged with murder but was acquitted on the grounds that the child was severely handicapped and that the parents had rejected the child. All the evidence given at the trial suggested that this was an appropriate way to deal with a handicapped baby.

Sometimes David might feel that he may as well support the idea of an abortion because even if the child was born, it might be legally disposed of in some way.

Infanticide, which was common in England before this century, was related to the lack of support given to new mothers in difficulty, the absence of contraception and the high mortality rate among small children which in any case existed. The twentieth century Western world idea of the value of the child as an individual was something which was not yet accorded to a profoundly disordered child. David knows that some people would think that it would be better to be dead than disabled.

Different Points of View

In the discussion that has taken place so far, three different points of view on abortion appear to be represented.

Agnes

Agnes believes that she has a right to determine what happens to her own body and that the fetus is merely a part of her body. She finds it difficult to imagine that abortion could ever be wrong. She feels that it is her right to choose what happens to her and if she has become pregnant by accident and decides that she does not want to have the child, that is her business, and perfectly legal (as long as she can persuade the doctor that she would be unwell if thwarted in her desire). She thinks it is kinder to abort than bring unwanted babies into the world.

Colin

Colin has a very conservative point of view. He believes that abortion at any time from conception onwards is always wrong. It is not clear what he would think if Agnes's life was at risk because of her pregnancy. There are some people who hold views like his who would feel

that it is always better to let the mother die in order to
save the child. Colin thinks that the fetus has a right to
life, and would act to prevent its destruction in any way —
even if it were not his child: all fetuses are innocent and
vulnerable, deserving protection.

David

For the purpose of this discussion we will ascribe to David
a moderate view which says on the one hand that abortion
should not be entered into lightly but, on the other, that
it can sometimes be justified depending on when it takes
place and why it is being done. He might be concerned
about the effect upon Agnes of not terminating the pregnancy. There are tragic occasions when abortion must be
allowed to bring about a greater good. He would not
interfere if one of his friends wanted one, but he feels he
must not let it happen to his own child.

The nurse and the doctor

The position of the doctor is unique. As the person who
performs the operation or who refers a woman to the
clinic for the operation to be performed, a doctor actually
makes the decision. The doctor has to work within the
law, but has a certain amount of discretion in deciding
whether the legal requirements are fulfilled. Health care
professionals who have a moral objection to abortion can
refuse to look after patients in these circumstances, but
they have to make sure that the patient is looked after by
someone else. Nurses can give their managers advanced
warning of a conscientious objection, but are never
allowed to act in such a way as to endanger the life of the
mother. Emergency treatment should therefore always be
provided by a nurse, no matter what the condition of the
mother. In deciding whether or not to use the conscience

clause, a health care professional would have to think about the balance of rights. The mother has a legal right to have an abortion (if she satisfies the legal requirements). As it is stated in the *Infant Life (Preservation) Act* 1929, a newborn infant has a legal right to life. From a moral point of view, the health care professional has to decide at what stage the fetus becomes a child and starts having the rights that a child would have. On the face of it, the difference between a child inside the mother's womb and the child moments later outside the mother's womb represents a significant stage of development, but there are other equally significant changes which do not have the effect of changing the moral status of the individual, like the first breath, the first word or the Christening or naming ceremony.

This kind of argument is of no interest to Agnes. She feels that her right to do what she wants with her own body overrides anybody else's rights, such as the right of the father, the right of the fetus and the right of anyone else in society who objects to what she is doing.

Colin argues that there is a 'potential person' there in order to persuade Agnes that she should not destroy the child or the fetus. In some ways, however, this is a self-defeating argument for him. If what he wants to say is that abortion is never acceptable, he should leave it at that. If he starts to argue about abortion in relation to personhood, he may find himself defining the point at which a fetus becomes a person. As a result of that he may find that he has conceded that there is a stage of pregnancy, even if it is only a very early stage, during which, consistent with his moral point of view, it would be acceptable to destroy the conceptus.

We decided to give David a moderate point of view. David is the kind of person who believes that there are some circumstances in which it would be reasonable to destroy a fetus. However, because of his special interest in children with severe learning difficulties, he does not personally regard the lifestyle of severely disabled persons as sufficiently traumatic and appalling to justify killing them before they are born. In some ways his is a quite unusually moderate position, because most people who hold the position that abortion is sometimes justified have quite clear views about what kind of life they think is not worth living. When you think about yourself and imagine those things which you hold dear, you may gain some insight as to what you personally would regard as a fate worse than death. For some athletic people, being physically handicapped might seem an intolerable burden. For people who enjoy an intellectual life, it may well seem that impaired capacity to reason would be unbearable for them. Things always get difficult when you start to try to estimate the value of someone else's life to them and their families, and how they value their own faculties.

Philosophers

The philosophical issues about abortion often cover three major areas.

Firstly, a definition is sought as to what makes something a person. The second point is whether is it intrinsically wrong to destroy potential persons. Thirdly, philosophy tries to clarify at what point in development a human being becomes a person and is not merely a potential person.

The philosopher Michael Tooley (1983) supports abortion on the grounds that a fetus is not a person. What makes something a person? A 'person' is usually thought of as a human being. When you think about why you regard your mother but not your cat as a person, it may be to do with the fact that your mother has some special qualities that a human being has. As well as being a member of the species, she can also walk and talk and reason. These are among the things that make a human special. We can say about a monkey that can do tricks and communicate that it is 'almost human'. If you are unfortunate enough to see your mother go into a decline and suffer from dementia, you might hear yourself and members of the family say that 'she's not the *person* she used to be'. If she was so ill that she reached a vegetative state, did not walk, talk, move or recognise anybody or have any kind of memory, you might say that she is scarcely a person at all. But she is still human, you cannot change that, even though you cannot relate to her as a person any more. Some people are quite comfortable with the idea that when human beings reach that state, their life is of no value to them any more and they ought to be allowed to die. They would not think of this as murder because it is not killing a person, but rather putting a human being out of his or her misery.

Comparisons are often made between the condition of the human being at the end of life and the condition of a human being soon after birth. In both cases communication is difficult, individuals are unable to fend for themselves, and it is difficult to know what they feel about themselves, or whether they have any meaningful internal life. Someone who would justify allowing a dependent old person to die, would probably not allow a newborn baby to die, because that baby is regarded as having *potential* and it is hoped that it will grow up to have all the qualities that we would expect of a human person.

The fetus in the uterus has some of the distinguishing marks that would be identified with personhood. It looks like a person. It is hard if you look at a photograph or if you find a fetus in the bedpan after a termination not to wonder whether, in any sense, this is a person that is now being disposed of.

As was seen from the historical account, it was believed in the past that someone became a person only when their body was inhabited by a soul. The legal distinctions that were made between early and late abortions suggest that the fetus was accorded some of the rights of personhood at the time when quickening took place. That is why the punishments for an abortion after that time were more akin to the punishments for murder.

Philosophers will have long discussions about what it is that constitutes persons and therefore what it is we have to do to show respect for persons. Tooley says that the fetus has no right to life because it is not a person. This has been questioned by Rosalind Hursthouse (1987). In reply she says that it is not morally acceptable to kill non-persons — consider Martians. When she criticised Tooley, Hursthouse pointed out a fault in his logic. He appears to be saying that it is wrong to kill a person, but the fact that someone is not a person makes killing them acceptable. Hursthouse argues that from a strictly logical point of view that is wrong, and she provides ample proof for her position. She gives the example of a Martian, saying that because this extra-terrestrial creature cannot possibly be a human being does not give us a justification for killing it. Intuitively that seems right. Anything that could communicate and move about would be interesting and valuable from a scientific, educational and entertainment point of view and therefore should be preserved. If, however, we discovered that Martians were highly nutritious, there might be some justification for farming them and feeding them to the starving millions of humans who are already on this earth. If they are living things but not human, we owe no more or less loyalty to them than we do to the animals that already share our planet with us.

Depending on your views, this could merely be an argument for vegetarianism. Nevertheless, these two philosophers are trying to work out what we ought to do and coming to very different conclusions. The ethics of nursing is concerned with what is right. The nurse has to take seriously the feelings of all the people involved. The nurse will therefore have to try to understand the differing values of the people who are involved in this case.

In his book on ethics for nurses, Richard Rowson (1990) describes 'the basic elements in moral thinking'.

> Morally important aspects of actions are: 1. When actions express attitudes to people . . . 2. When actions have certain qualities that make the actions right or wrong in themselves . . . 3. When actions are likely to affect certain people in certain ways . . . 4. When actions are done from certain motives . . . 5. When actions are natural or unnatural . . . 6. When actions agree with God's will or go against it . . .

When the nurse is thinking about whether it is right or wrong for Agnes to have an abortion, these six categories could be taken into account.

1. Actions expressing attitudes to people

The idea of autonomy is central to the UKCC *Code of Professional Conduct* (1992). The thing that distinguishes a 'person' is the fact that he or she is a rational human being. Rational human beings can never use the defence that they were obeying orders if they do something that is morally wrong. Conscientious objection in war time and conscientious objection to abortion by health care workers recognise this fact. It may also mean, from one point of view, that the person who believes a law is morally wrong must do everything possible to get that law changed. People may believe that breaking the law ('civil disobedience') is not just acceptable but in fact necessary in the face of bad laws. The American Anti-Abortion Campaign 'Operation Rescue' has used extreme measures to, in their view, rescue the innocent. They block the entrances to abortion clinics and attract attention to themselves by going to jail and refusing to give their names in the courts.

If you think that a mature person has the right to self-determination, showing respect for Agnes might include allowing her, unhindered, to have an abortion. The dilemma comes if, like Colin, you believe the fetus is also a person, and therefore it must be allowed to live in order to show it respect. There are times when persons are not allowed full expression of autonomy. There are times when we say that patients must have restrictions placed upon them for their own good, for example when they are confused or mentally ill. If David respects Agnes's position as a person, he may attempt to influence her decision to have the abortion by rational argument, but would go no further in attempting to stop her having the abortion. Colin might go further. The position of any nurse is that, when acting as a nurse, you are not allowed to dissuade someone from having an abortion but you are allowed to refuse to take part as long as the woman has no immediate emergency needs.

Bearing in mind that the UKCC *Code of Professional Conduct* requires that a nurse act in a professional way at all times, do you think that a nurse could be removed from the Register for taking part in activities such as 'Operation Rescue'?

2. Certain actions are right or wrong in themselves

This is known as the Deontological view. One example of the Deontological view is that taking life is always wrong. Because life is a good thing, destroying it is in itself a bad thing.

This is the point of view that Colin would probably hold. Looking back at the section on contraception, one can see that Colin may well think that any form of contraception is bad. It has been argued in the past that masturbation is a sin because it means that potential human life is destroyed as semen that is not used for procreation is produced. This visible spilling of seed contributed to the general disapprobation in which male homosexual behaviour was held by the Church. The sin of homosexuality was thought to be one that women could not commit because there was no visible sin of the wasting of potential human life. The only way a woman could sin in this respect was by refusing to submit to her husband, by using contraceptives or by attempting to abort her fetus.

For Agnes the foundation of her morality may be that everyone's personal autonomy should be respected. She should have the right to control her body. For Colin the basic tenet of his moral belief might be that you always respect human life, and anything that damages human life is wrong in itself.

It has been argued by Dunstan and Sellar (1988) that selecting the sex of a child to be born is wrong in itself. They say that 'the calculation of personal preference for a child of one sex or the other diminishes the awe in which we stand before both'.

Do you think that an abortion would be wrong in itself because Agnes is interested in determining the sex of her children?

3. Morally right actions are those which are most useful in producing the best consequences for everyone

This is known as the Utilitarian view. It is probably closest to what David thinks. David does not have a strong view that abortion is always wrong. He can imagine situations in which abortion might bring about the best consequences, for example when it makes the mother unwell or she would be forced to continue with the pregnancy. The problem for David is that his assessment of the best consequences may not be the same as those of the others. Agnes might think that it is better to be dead than handicapped. Colin might think it is better to allow a fetus to live than to degrade the humanity of the mother by allowing her to have an abortion. The problem with David's point of view is that the outcome, which he cannot necessarily know about until afterwards, determines whether or not what was done was morally correct. So if David thinks that it is better that the child should not be born and Agnes becomes desperately ill and dies as a result of it, David's action is wrong. If David thinks that it is best that the child should be born and there is an outcome that gives rise to there being more evil in the world than there was before (for example, the child becomes a mass murderer), David's action is also wrong. Another problem with this is deciding at what stage you are going to stop the measure of the outcome of an action. There is a popular saying that everything will be the same in 100 years' time. When you weigh up the pluses and minuses of Agnes's little tragedy, it may not greatly add to or detract from the sum of good or evil for the human race.

Many of the problems of resource distribution that nurses wrestle with every day are solved using broadly Utilitarian principles. In deciding to make an equitable distribution of the health care resources that are available, health care professionals may be persuaded that the resources required by a profoundly handicapped person after birth are not being used in the best way. The 'quality–adjusted life year' (QALY) is a crude way of measuring the effectiveness of resources that are used in health care. Given that the life of the child is predicted to be short and unpleasant, it may well be that by using a QALY calculation one would decide that this life was not worth putting any resources into. It might even be decided that it is an economically fair action to abort the fetus before he starts being a drain on the system. A broad view of Utilitarianism would suggest that happiness is not always measured by the amount of health care resources that are spread around, and the emotional effect of abortion should be taken into account when making the equation; therefore, even if abortion were a fair solution from an economic point of view, it would not be justifiable if the amount of distress caused to the mother and other handicapped people was very great. It is difficult to know what to do for the best when there are a number of people who would be upset in different ways according to whether or not there were an abortion.

Do you think that Colin or David would be justified in saying that Agnes must have the child because they are prepared to overcome any of the subsequent difficulties that it might present?

4. Moral motivation is the concern to do the right actions and avoid the wrong ones

Although intention seems to be quite a simple concept, it is something about which philosophers have written many books and articles. As can be seen from the Roman Catholic analysis of abortion, a person can have a double intent when doing anything. The surgeon can remove the fallopian tube with the intention of removing a diseased tube or can remove the fallopian tube with the intent of terminating a pregnancy. If one of these is allowed and the other is not, the surgeon might claim that what is being done is permitted, and that the other consequence is not intended, and therefore the surgeon cannot be responsible for it. I might say that I cannot be responsible for your broken leg if you slip on a wet floor that I have just been washing in a hospital corridor, because my intention was to clean the floor, not to harm you. Nevertheless, from a common sense point of view, most people would agree that a wet floor in a public place should be signposted in some way in order to prevent accidents, and that the person who made the floor wet has a duty to make the hazard clear, and is responsible for any failure to do so.

The disconcerting thing about people who use their intentions as a justification for their actions alone, without reference to the outcome, is that one might imagine a situation in which you could *delude* yourself into thinking that you were doing things for one reason, but without any justification.

The road to hell, it is said, is paved with good intentions. Nevertheless, it has to be said that a person who is acting in a moral way must always be concerned about trying to do the right thing and avoiding the wrong thing. It has been suggested that if Agnes has an abortion because she does not want to have a male child, she has a bad motive. If she thinks the child should never be born because of its severe handicap and the likelihood of a distressing life, you might think that she has a good motive. This would be supported by the law, which allows severe handicap as a justification for abortion. But Colin and David both have good motives for persuading her to have the child. David thinks that having the child would be the best consequence because he would be able to take care of it and keep it happy, and an abortion can be harmful. He also believes that if he cannot persuade Agnes of this, it is better for her to have the abortion. Colin believes that whatever else happens, Agnes should not have the abortion because it would degrade her.

What do you think Agnes's motives are?

5. Acting in accordance with nature

One of the best examples of this kind of thinking is when we consider the arguments around resuscitating people towards the end of life. Some people think that it is better to let someone die naturally rather than to interfere with them and mobilise the entire resources of a team of health care professionals just to keep someone alive for a short period of time. To allow natural death seems the right thing to do and the unnatural prolongation of life seems like a bad thing. As Rowson says, the view that 'unnatural' acts are wrong obviously relies on being able to make a distinction between natural and unnatural acts.

Any action that is taken can be seen as interfering with nature. Unless your action has some effect, you can hardly be said to have acted. In science fiction stories, time travellers are urged not to interfere with what is going on in the time and space, to avoid altering the course of nature. Any action, however trivial, can have effects which will influence the world they enter. In real life – by harnessing energy, cultivating plants, using birth control etc. — we in many ways continuously interfere with nature. It is possible to argue that some actions 'help' nature. The midwife who helps the mother in a difficult labour may prevent the death of either mother or child. She may use natural methods to assist childbirth, but without her, the mother and child would naturally die. Other things seem 'against' nature, for example surrogate pregnancies or organ transplants.

Other people claim that there are certain things that are in accordance with 'human' nature. Certain kinds of behaviour may be labelled 'inhuman'. Standing by and allowing the mother and child to die might seem 'inhuman'. The natural instinct of many people is to help and sustain others. It may also be natural to behave in a way that serves your own best interest. The abortion, Agnes thinks, is in her own best interest. Colin is concerned about the interest of the child. One of the arguments put forward by 'Life' (the anti-abortion campaign) against the woman's right to choose is that the child is a third party with an interest that must be represented. It is natural that someone might attempt to defend the child. The very idea of abortion gives rise to what Dunstan and Sellar (1988) call 'moral repugnance'. They describe an internal sensation of distaste which is natural to them in the face of certain ideas and actions. Some ideas of distaste are learned, like a horror of dirt, or a reluctance to eat certain foods, such as insects. There may be some groups who find eating flies satisfying but this is a matter of taste, not ethics.

The idea of doing the right thing by doing what is in one's nature is shared by Eastern philosophers, and the fact that there are many moral tenets which are common to all ethical systems would indicate that there is something that is natural for human beings to want to believe.

Is it unnatural for a woman to want to have an abortion?

6. Right actions are those which are in agreement with God's will

As has been seen in the section on religious beliefs and abortion, there is no general agreement about what is the will of God in this matter. The Christian religions have reached differing conclusions from the same source material. Women within the Church have argued that the men who have interpreted the scriptures have done so in a way that is influenced more by their gender and social roles than the will of God. None of the people around Agnes has expressed a belief in God or a particular religious conviction. If someone were to try to persuade her that it was God's will that the child should live, she might reply in a number of ways. Firstly, she might say that she has read the Bible and there is nothing there that suggests God would disapprove. Secondly, she might say that she has prayed and thought and she feels sure that it is God's will that she should not be a mother. The fact that the child is male and handicapped is evidence — God has made it easy for her to obtain an abortion.

There are not many role models for the religious woman who wants to avoid motherhood. A child in the Bible is often seen as a gift from God — the ultimate example of this being the Immaculate Conception. Nevertheless, in Third World countries where control of fertility is problematic, even priests take a supportive line when women seek abortion.

What should a nurse do when faced with a patient who has a different view of the will of God?

Legislation

The Offences Against the Person Act 1861
The Infant Life (Preservation) Act 1929
The Abortion Act 1986
The Human Fertilisation and Embryology Act 1990
The Abortion Regulations 1991

R v Bourne (1938)
R v Arthur (1981)
RCN   v DHSS (1981)
Janaway v Salford Health Authority (1988)
C v S (1988)

References

Dunstan, G. and Sellar, M. (1988) *The Status of the Human Embryo*. London, Kings Fund Publishing.
Hursthouse, R. (1987) *Beginning Lives*. Oxford, Blackwell.
Rowson, R. (1990) *An Introduction to Ethics for Nurses*. London, Scutari Press.
Tooley, M. (1983) *Abortion and Infanticide*. Oxford, Clarendon Press.

UKCC (1992) *Code of Professional Conduct* (3rd Edn). London, UKCC.

Further Reading

Chervenak, F.A. and McCullough, L.B. (1991) Respect for the autonomy of the pregnant woman in surrogacy agreements: an elaboration of a fundamental ethical concern. *Women's Health Issues*, **1**(3) Summer, pp. 143–4.

Dawson, K. (1987) Fertilisation and moral status, a scientific perspective. *The Journal of Medical Ethics*, **13**: 173–8.

Downie, R.S. and Calman, K.C. (1987) *Healthy Respect: Ethics in Health Care*. London, Faber.

Gates, E.A. (1990) Maternal choice, will it work both ways? *Women's Health Issues*, **1**(1), Fall, pp. 25–7.

Greenwood, V. and Young, J. (1976) *Abortion in Demand*. London, Pluto Press.

Hall, M.H. (1990) Changes in the law on abortion won't produce radical changes (practice). *BMJ*, **301**, 17 Nov: 1109.

Kennedy, I. (1988) *Treat Me Right: Essays in Medical Law and Ethics*. Oxford, Clarendon Press.

Knapman, P. and West, I. (1989) *Medicine and the Law*. Oxford, Heinemann Medical Books.

Potts, M., Diggory, P. and Peel J. (1977) *Abortion*. Cambridge, Cambridge University Press.

Scarisbrick, J. (1971) *What's Wrong with Abortion* (this booklet is one of a series produced by LIFE).

CHAPTER 2

Organ Transplantation

Davina Gilbert
Jennifer Iliffe and **Pamela Swan**
Verena Tschudin

Organ transplantation has only been possible for a comparatively short time in the history of medicine. In that time it has acquired a prestige which is astonishing when compared to the numbers of cases actually involved.

Only practices at the boundaries of the possible are questioned as ethical. Most transplants are still in that category. Indeed, the two main types of transplant discussed in this chapter (kidney and heart transplants) show this clearly by the difficulties which the three authors describe as paramount. The difficulties of communication highlighted in the section on kidney transplants are certainly not unique to just one situation. The emotional and psychological problems considered by the authors of the section concerning heart transplants also show that ethics is first and foremost about listening to each other. For this reason the authors raise questions which challenge the readers first to listen to themselves and hear their own values and beliefs. With this knowledge they then need to find ways to make themselves heard.

Kidney Transplantation

In this section, some of the ethical and moral dilemmas facing nurses who care for renal transplant patients will

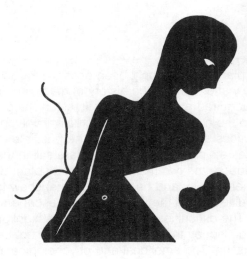

be discussed. Case histories, the identities in which have been changed, will be included relating to the following topics:

- Tissue matching.
- Waiting list criteria.
- Live related donors.
- Infection risks.
- Graft survival versus patient wellbeing.
- Errors in clinical practice.
- Patient information.
- Consent.

Renal nurses need to consider the ethical and moral dilemmas relating to diseases of the kidney for the following reasons:

- The UKCC *Code of Professional Conduct* (1992) requires nurses to safeguard the wellbeing and interests of their patients.
- Caring for patients with chronic renal failure demands that nurses build close relationships with their patients in order to provide holistic nursing care.
- Current clinical practice does not always give enough consideration to the physical and psychological wellbeing of renal patients; nurses are therefore responsible for much of that care.

Many of the issues discussed in this chapter relate to problems of communication between medical and nursing staff. This is not in itself an ethical problem, but when it affects patients' physical and psychological wellbeing, it must be considered as one. In order to deal with the issues arising from current practice, nurses must involve themselves fully in the whole process of transplantation and challenge any practices which they believe are not in the best interest of their patients.

The majority of problems that nurses encounter result from the widespread opinion that successful kidney transplantation is considered to be the most effective treatment for patients suffering from end stage renal failure:

- For the patient, transplantation is seen as a straightforward solution which will provide restored health and freedom from the constraints of dialysis treatment.
- For the hospital business manager, successful kidney transplantation is the most cost effective treatment as it reduces the demand for limited hospital resources.
- For the medical and nursing staff, successful kidney transplantation has come to be seen as essential. It enables them to take on the increasing numbers of new patients for dialysis treatment and to provide a

better quality of life for patients with chronic renal failure.

For these and other local or personal reasons, a great deal of effort is put into promoting kidney transplantation as the best treatment for all kidney patients. However, although a renal transplant provides the best substitute for kidneys which have failed, the process is not risk free nor is it guaranteed to be successful.

Tissue matching

Before a kidney transplant takes place, the donor and recipient are matched in the following categories:

- Blood group compatibility.
- Human leucocyte antigen compatibility.
- Cross matching and mixed lymphocyte culture.

Tissue matching is a very complex subject, an exact match only being found between identical twins. Tissue matching for kidney transplantation is concerned with finding a good enough match between donor and recipient that the graft is not rejected. Because of the complexity of the matching procedure, it is impossible to lay down exact criteria for acceptable matching. Clinical judgement is ultimately used to try to ensure that the best possible matches are made.

A national transplant scheme known as the UK Transplant Support Service (UKTSS) coordinates the distribution of donated organs. The scheme operates on a sharing basis. Each participating hospital registers potential recipients' blood groups, tissue types and acceptable matching criteria on the central computer database. **Beneficial matching** is the term used when all the criteria for the best possible match have been met (UK Transplant Support Service 1990). Hospitals which belong to the scheme must donate at least one kidney from each pair retrieved locally. When an organ becomes available, the best matched recipient in the country is identified and the appropriate hospital notified.

However, some large hospitals may donate more kidneys to the scheme than they receive. For this reason, they may choose not to belong and to operate on a local basis only. This enables them to use all the kidneys that they retrieve to carry out transplants within their own patient population.

The advantage to hospitals of belonging to the UKTSS scheme is that their patients have a greater chance of receiving beneficially matched kidneys with a lower risk of graft rejection during the first year (UK Transplant Support Service 1990). This increases their potential for long term survival. However, patients may wait longer for a transplant because they are on a national waiting list.

The advantage to hospitals in opting out of the UKTSS scheme is that patients have a much higher chance of being transplanted within a shorter period because they are on a local waiting list. However, they are less likely to receive a beneficially matched kidney. This may reduce potential for long term survival.

This raises some ethical issues. Renal nurses are aware that kidneys retrieved locally may have a poorer match than those obtained through UKTSS. They often have to deal with situations where they know that a patient is to receive a kidney which is not beneficially matched. In these cases, the risk of graft rejection is increased and the wellbeing of the patient may be jeopardised.

- Carol, aged 33, was the mother of two young children, aged 9 and 11. She had received two kidney transplants, the first of which failed in the immediate post-operative period. The second functioned for six years, gradually deteriorating in the 18 months before it failed.

Carol was then re-established on Continuous Ambulatory Peritoneal Dialysis (CAPD). Her main problem was lack of energy which made it difficult to look after her children and to carry out her dialysis treatment. She had a good relationship with the dialysis nurses and discussed her problems openly. She desperately wanted another transplant to give her freedom and the energy to cope with bringing up her children.

After two years, a cadaver kidney, with which Carol's tissue type and blood group were considered compatible, became available for transplantation. However, the renal nurses knew that the kidney had been locally retrieved and that the level of matching was comparatively low. They were concerned that, as this would be Carol's third transplant, it ought to be beneficially matched so that it would have a higher potential for long-term survival. They were also aware that the surgical procedure for transplantation becomes progressively more difficult with each operation, increasing the risk of failure.

In this case, although Carol was aware of the increased surgical risks, she decided to receive the transplant. The renal nurses did not try to influence Carol's choice. After the operation, she suffered several episodes of rejection which were treated and eventually controlled. Carol's transplant, although functioning reasonably well, will always require high doses of immunosuppressive therapy to maintain its function. This increases the risk of debilitating side effects. It is unlikely that this kidney will survive for more than a few years. Carol is likely to be back on dialysis before she is 40.

Should the nurses have tried to influence Carol's decision? They knew that she was desperate for another transplant and that she was not receptive to any ideas which may have appeared to be negative. The UKCC *Code of Professional Conduct* (1992) requires nurses to safeguard the interests and wellbeing of their patients. In this instance, should the nurses have prepared Carol better for the decision she had to make long before a kidney became available for her? Since they had many of the medical criteria to hand, should they also have been prepared to discuss their fears for the survival of this transplant with the medical team?

Waiting list criteria

The demand for kidneys for transplantation has risen steadily over the last 10 years and greatly exceeds the supply. In June 1991 potential recipients numbered 3342, while during the six month period from January to June 1991, only 758 cadaver transplants and 27 live related donor transplants were performed (UKTSS Bulletin 1991).

At each hospital, a number of renal patients are considered to be ready to receive a transplant. When a kidney becomes available which could be transplanted into more than one patient, a decision has to be made regarding which patient should be offered the kidney. The highest priority is given to any patient who is on the last possible access site for dialysis and who will die if a suitable kidney is not found. If there are no high priority patients, other factors need to be considered when making the decision. For example, the choice may be between a patient who has already had a transplant which has failed and a patient who has been waiting for several years on dialysis never having been offered a transplant. The choice may be between a young disabled person and an older person with a family to support.

Since the demand for kidney transplants greatly exceeds the supply, who should be given priority and what should the criteria be? The renal nurse may well have a view on this, but in many cases she will not be consulted, as the following case study illustrates.

- Before his kidney transplant, Tom, aged 20, had no experience of dialysis treatment. After receiving a transplant from his brother, he suffered life-threatening complications resulting in the removal of the transplanted kidney.

Confronted with the urgent need for dialysis treatment, Tom insisted that he would prefer haemodialysis to CAPD. Attempts to create permanent vascular access for haemodialysis were unsuccessful. Consequently, Tom had to start CAPD.

In order to persuade Tom to accept CAPD treatment, medical staff told him that this would be for a temporary period only. He would be a priority on the waiting list for a cadaver transplant. The nurses knew that Tom was not a priority for transplantation because his CAPD treatment was working successfully. However, they felt that they could not disillusion Tom because his recent trauma had destroyed all his confidence in the hospital system. He had become depressed and uncommunicative. His subsequent CAPD training period was fraught with difficulties. His conviction that CAPD was temporary and that his only hope was a second transplant made it almost impossible for the nurses to help him to adjust to his life on CAPD.

After three months on the waiting list, just as Tom was beginning to adjust to his circumstances, he was called for a second transplant. The nurses had already voiced their opinion that Tom was not psychologically ready to face the trauma of another operation and that he should only be considered for transplant if the available kidney were a beneficial match. The nurses were not consulted when the decision was made to give Tom the second transplant, which was not beneficially matched.

The post-operative period was once again traumatic and life threatening, with severe rejection episodes. During this period, Tom was so distressed that he was unable to talk about his condition or to face the possibility of losing a second transplanted kidney. After 12 weeks, the kidney finally functioned and Tom no longer needed CAPD. However, the prognosis for the survival of the kidney was poor because of the post-operative trauma.

In telling Tom that he was a priority for a second

transplant, the medical staff were trying to compensate for the failure of the first transplant. Did the nurses acquiesce in misleading Tom because they did not know how he would react to knowing that he was not a priority, or because they did not want him to lose even more confidence in the renal staff? In acting as patient advocates, nurses should have been prepared to persist in their opposition to a non-beneficially matched transplant for Tom.

The nurses had recommended that Tom should only receive a kidney with a high level of tissue matching. They had also recommended that Tom should not be made a priority on the waiting list. In the event, the nurses' recommendations were not taken into consideration. Fortunately, Tom's transplanted kidney eventually functioned. The injunction on nurses, to be responsible for their patients' wellbeing, means also that they need to challenge channels of communication and medical paternalism.

Live related donors

The live related donation of organs is protected by the Unrelated Live Transplant Regulatory Authority (ULTRA). This organisation was set up in 1990 following a much publicised incident where a transplant operation was carried out using a kidney purchased from a Turkish man. The purpose of ULTRA is to prevent the sale of organs for transplantation and to ensure that transplants are not carried out between live donors and recipients who are not closely genetically related.

If a patient with renal failure has a healthy parent or sibling who wishes to donate a kidney, then a full medical assessment is carried out to establish compatibility. The psychological assessment and preparation of both donor and recipient are equally important.

Officially, medical staff do not ask patients if they have

relatives who would consider becoming live related donors. However, in practice, patients are often asked this question, or ask it themselves. In general, there are few guidelines as to how and when such an interview should be conducted. Patients are often asked at a time when they are only beginning to learn about the impact of their renal failure. This can be very distressing for patients who may feel under pressure to provide a donor. In addition, it may cause conflict and anxiety within their families. Patients may not always know who to approach for more advice and information.

- John, aged 30, had been on dialysis for 18 months. His sister Janet, aged 35, was the most suitable kidney donor out of five siblings. Janet was under a lot of pressure from her parents and other siblings to donate her kidney. She felt obliged to consider donating her kidney so that John would be free from dialysis but she was most reluctant to do so. She felt that her young children were her first responsibility. She was also frightened of the surgery involved.

  In this case, the nurse who had been caring for John for several months had to play an important role in counselling both Janet and John. The nurse decided to provide support for Janet's decision and ensured that the medical staff were fully aware of her reluctance to proceed.

In supporting Janet, the nurse was instrumental in denying John the chance of a live related kidney transplant. It was also important for the nurse to maintain a good relationship with John throughout this difficult period. Could she have done more to help Janet, John and the whole family to come to terms with Janet's decision? Perhaps the involvement of a trained counsellor, who would have the time and skills to address the family's varying needs and emotions, might have been appropriate.

- Mary had been on dialysis for 12 months. Her sister Jane was a suitable donor who was very keen to donate a kidney.

The sisters were part of an extremely close knit and supportive family.

After the successful transplant operation, Jane was nursed in a surgical ward some distance from the transplant unit. She experienced complications during her recovery period which prevented her from visiting her sister in the renal ward, although she was very anxious about her. Jane felt that she had been pushed to one side after her kidney had been removed and that no-one was interested in her recovery. She said that the owner of her body might just as well have stayed at home.

Mary's recovery was deeply and unforgettably distressing to her. She felt upset, guilty and very anxious about Jane's problems, particularly as their only contact with one another was via a third party, often a busy nurse.

In this case, nursing staff could have presented a strong case, supported by their professional Code, for nursing these patients in the same ward. Such a holistic approach would have alleviated much of the anxiety experienced by both Jane and Mary. However, in other circumstances, where a live related transplant kidney fails, or where serious complications occur, nursing both donor and recipient in the same ward may be detrimental to the recovery of both, as the suffering of one affects the other.

- Mohammed was a young student from the Middle East studying in the UK. His whole family lived abroad.

  When it was realised that he was progressing towards end stage renal failure, the medical staff decided that a live related donor transplant would be the best option for him because dialysis treatment in his own country was limited and costly.

  Mohammed's mother was a suitable donor. When she arrived in the UK further medical investigations revealed mild hypertension and a small kidney stone. Mohammed's mother spoke no English. Medical and nursing discussions with her were difficult because an interpreter was not always

available. The nurses were concerned because they did not
think that Mohammed's mother should have been
considered as a kidney donor because of her hypertension
and kidney stone. It was also unclear to them how much
information she had been given and how much she had
understood. Despite the medical complications, the medical
and surgical teams performed the transplant, removing the
kidney stone during the operation.

Three years later, the transplanted kidney failed and
Mohammed started haemodialysis in the UK. The state of
his mother's health is unknown as she returned home shortly
after the transplant.

In this case the nurses should perhaps have expressed their
concerns on the following grounds:

• The health and wellbeing of the donor and recipient
  were at risk.
• Both mother and son had received insufficient information and counselling to make the decision.
• The mother's decision to donate her kidney may
  have been so strongly influenced by cultural and
  moral pressures that she was prepared to sacrifice her
  own health.
• Further investigation into Mohammed's family may
  have revealed a more suitable related donor.

Infection risks

Cytomegalovirus (CMV) is one of the herpes group of
viruses. Although it does not produce significant disease
in healthy adults, it can cause severe pneumonitis in
immunocompromised patients. This can sometimes be
fatal.

Studies of the prevalence of antibody against CMV in the
general population show that infection of this virus is
widespread and usually inapparent. Depending

on the socio-economic condition of the population, the prevalence of antibodies in adults ranges from 40 per cent to 100 per cent. (Mandell et al 1990)

CMV can be detected by a routine blood test. All kidneys that become available for transplantation are tested for CMV status. However, at the moment current practice does not always take into consideration the CMV status of the recipient.

The implications of transplanting a CMV-positive kidney into a CMV-negative patient are that:

- the potential for life-threatening infection is increased, particularly during the immediate post-operative period when the immunosuppressive drugs are introduced in high doses;
- the patient will become CMV positive and will always be at risk of developing infections because of the immunosuppressive therapy.

The Department of Health circular on patient consent to examination (1990) states that:

> where tissues or organs are to be transplanted, the recipient should be informed at the time when consent to operation is obtained of the small, but unavoidable risk of the transplant being infected.

It would seem obvious that the recipients should be given the information on the CMV status of the donor kidney, thereby allowing them to make their own decision on whether to proceed with the transplant operation. However, is it reasonable to expect that every patient considering a transplant is able to make an objective decision to refuse such a kidney? Patients' thoughts are likely to be focused on life without dialysis. Is it fair then to force them to consider additional risks? The issue of informed consent needs to be considered here.

Graft survival versus patient wellbeing

The survival of any transplanted kidney is of the utmost importance to the patient and the medical and nursing staff. The majority of patients are willing to accept a great deal of stress and pain without question if they believe it will ensure the survival of their new kidney transplant.

If surgical or medical complications occur, there is a danger that the renal team could impose on the patient, and assume without question, the belief that any patient would put the survival of his kidney before anything else.

- Sandra was a full-time dance teacher who coped extremely well with CAPD. She turned down her first offer of a kidney transplant because she could not take time off work. After two years on CAPD, Sandra was offered a second kidney, which she accepted.

  After the transplant, she suffered severe graft rejection and thrombosis of the renal vein. During the rejection episode, Sandra nearly died. She knew that her condition was critical and confided in the nurses that she wanted the transplanted kidney to be removed. It appeared to her that the survival of the kidney was more important to the medical staff than her own life.

  The nurses voiced their opinion that Sandra had suffered enough and that the transplanted kidney should be removed. However, the medical team felt that there was still a small chance that the kidney would survive.

  Over the next two weeks, Sandra was subjected to numerous invasive tests and every attempt was made to save the transplanted kidney. Finally, the medical team decided to remove the kidney.

  Afterwards Sandra was transferred to a medical ward. She felt very bitter and believed that her immediate removal from the transplant ward indicated that the renal staff regarded her as a failure and were no longer interested in her wellbeing. She felt that she had suffered a lot of unnecessary pain and trauma.

In this case, as patient advocates, should the nurses have persevered in trying to influence the medical team's decision on Sandra's behalf? The medical team did not take into account the wishes of the patient, possibly feeling that her critical state of health did not enable her to make an objective decision. The medical decision needs to be balanced by the decisions or recommendations and wishes of all concerned.

- David was just adjusting to life on CAPD when a cadaver kidney became available.

    The level of tissue matching was comparatively low. The post-operative period was traumatic and David was kept in hospital for a period of three months. During this time, he suffered severe rejection episodes and life-threatening complications which necessitated nursing him in the intensive care unit.

    David had to continue with dialysis treatment (CAPD) but, because of his poor state of health, the dialysis was inefficient. He showed obvious signs of fluid overload, which put considerable strain on his heart, and his blood pressure was difficult to control. He also developed a pleural effusion. A kidney biopsy showed severe rejection which meant that it was unlikely to function well.

    At this point, the nurses voiced their opinion that the immunosuppressive therapy should be discontinued to prevent further damage to David's health and wellbeing. They felt that David needed to come to terms with the fact that the kidney was probably going to fail. The medical team actively pursued all avenues of treatment to save the kidney.

    David did not want to give up hope that the kidney would function. He did not question the medical team's decisions although he became withdrawn and depressed. He was unable to consider the possibility of the kidney failing. Eventually, after three and a half months, the kidney started to function and David is now able to lead a normal life.

In this case, the nurses were concerned that the survival

of the transplanted kidney was being pursued at too great a cost to David's physical and psychological wellbeing. David was determined not to consider the possibility of his graft failing. How should the nurses have handled this conflict between acting according to their Code of Conduct and acting in accordance with David's wishes? Formal and informal discussions and meetings, case conferences, and possibly calling on a third party to referee meetings, are all feasible and practical ways forward.

Errors in clinical practice

In any discipline, despite strict policy and protocol, errors occasionally occur. When this happens, the patient should be informed as soon as possible.

How much information should the patient be given regarding any error which has been made? What should the nurse do if she feels that insufficient or inaccurate information has been given to a patient? What should nurses do if they think that errors are being covered up; should they blow the whistle?

- Ashok, aged 55, was unemployed and had been on dialysis treatment for six years. During this period, he had received two unsuccessful kidney transplants.

  Some time after the second failed transplant, it was discovered that Ashok was blood group 'B' despite a report in his medical case notes stating that he was blood group 'O'. Both kidney transplants had been performed on the assumption that he was blood group 'O'. In addition, the second transplant had a cold ischaemic time of 48 hours. This is the length of time that the donor kidney is stored prior to transplant; the maximum acceptable time is 36 hours (Green 1983). The kidney subsequently failed after six days.

  Both transplant failures could not be totally attributed to the clinical error of incorrect blood group documentation because they were both ABO compatible. However, the failure of the second transplant was most likely due to the lengthy cold ischaemic time prior to transplantation.

Ashok was not told about the error. His English was poor and his understanding of his treatment and condition was limited. He was not in good health and the medical staff felt that the knowledge of these errors would have been detrimental to his wellbeing.

Ashok's nurses felt that he had a right to know that errors had been made. They recognised that he would need a lot of help and support in understanding the nature of the errors and his rights as a patient. However, no nurse was prepared to reveal the errors without sanction from senior medical staff for fear of being reprimanded. They were also uncertain about the legal implications of doing so. Should the nurses have escalated the problem through the nursing hierarchy? This has become a thorny topic and no clear guidelines are available to nurses at present. If they take action alone, they risk losing their jobs. Group action may carry more weight, but this is lengthier and a spokesperson is needed.

- Helen, aged 32, was a diabetic who had both legs amputated above the knee. With the aid of artificial limbs, Helen was reasonably mobile. She had two young children and was separated from her husband.

  A kidney became available for transplantation on the second day of her CAPD training programme. She was totally unprepared for this event, as she thought that kidney transplantation would occur some time in the future. However, she realised that she was lucky to receive a kidney so quickly and was keen to have the transplant. The nurse responsible for Helen's CAPD training was not consulted before the transplant took place.

  On completion of the transplant operation the medical staff discovered that a serious error had been made. Helen's blood group was 'O' Negative while the transplanted kidney's blood group was 'A' Positive. Helen's blood group had

been listed incorrectly on the hospital's transplant list.
However, her blood group was correctly documented in
her medical case notes.

When the mistake was realised, attempts were made to
prevent rejection by performing plasma exchange. This
treatment was unsuccessful and an urgent operation was
necessary to remove the transplanted kidney.

When Helen's condition improved, she was told of the
mistake. Although her initial reaction was subdued, Helen
lost all confidence in the nurses, doctors and anyone
connected with the hospital. She was re-established on
CAPD but maintains the minimum of contact with the unit.
She does not want to have another transplant.

The nurse in charge of Helen's CAPD training felt that the
error might have been prevented had she been involved in
the decision to perform the transplant. She was already
familiar with Helen's blood group. Could she have been
more assertive in ensuring that she was involved in
decisions relating to her patient? Mistakes are costly in
terms of confidence and money. Being a patient's advocate is not only worthwhile, but often life-saving.

Patient information

It is important that the patient considering renal transplantation is adequately informed about the risks involved.

In some hospitals, a transplant coordinator or nurse is
available to counsel and support patients contemplating
either live related or cadaver kidney transplantation.
Unfortunately this is not the case in all hospitals, with the
result that the provision of information is left to the clinic
doctor, or to the nurse on the transplant ward immediately prior to the operation.

When a kidney becomes available for transplantation,
there is little time to spend on counselling and lengthy
explanations of treatment. Therefore, it is essential that

this information has been discussed with the patient well before the operation.

It is accepted practice in nursing to give information to patients regarding their treatment. However, in the case of kidney transplantation, it is difficult to know just how much information should be given to patients without causing unnecessary stress and anxiety. In addition, a nurse who tries to prepare patients to face difficulties or problems may be seen by medical staff as obstructive, difficult or interfering because patients' anxieties may be increased.

- Pat, aged 28, had been established on CAPD for six months. She was a quiet, shy and withdrawn person who lived alone.
  Pat had a successful kidney transplant. Her recovery period was traumatic as she was unprepared for the invasive procedures, drug therapy and frequent follow-up care required. She found the kidney biopsy and endoscopy particularly painful and frightening. Pat said that she thought that having a kidney transplant would be like taking her car for an MOT, a straightforward procedure completed in a day.

In this case, how could the nurses have established that Pat was adequately prepared for the transplant? Pat's recovery period could have been less stressful if she had received holistic care which included appropriate counselling and information from the nurses and doctors.

Consent

Correctly managed, knowledge of the truth can be positive and should be every patient's right. (Fletcher and Shrigley 1991)

Every surgical and medical procedure requires the patient's consent. Very often this consent is based on the patient's trust and confidence in the doctors and nurses involved. Consent *should* be based on the truth.

To what extent should patients be involved in decisions regarding complex health issues, such as the removal of a failing kidney transplant or the acceptance of a kidney with a low tissue match? How much should medical and nursing staff influence patients' decisions?

Although 'truth' and 'honesty' are not mentioned in the nurses' Code of Conduct, they are the basis of holistic nursing practice. The information which a patient can accept at any one time has to be judged on an individual basis. Nurses are often able to establish a close relationship with the patient which may better qualify them to assess the amount of information that a patient can absorb. This places a very heavy responsibility on the nurse. Therefore, it is essential that nurses work closely with all members of the multidisciplinary team to ensure that their patients are given truthful information regarding their treatment. In addition, their patients will require continuing support to help them to understand the information and to make informed decisions.

Conclusion

The pressures to perform kidney transplantation can build up an irresistible momentum. These pressures are not solely governed by a concern for patient welfare. They include:

- increasing numbers of patients with chronic renal failure;
- financial pressures;
- patient demand;
- the progression of medical science.

However, nurses are aware that transplantation may not always be in the best interests of patients and their families. This situation gives rise to a number of moral and ethical dilemmas for nurses. Since their Code of Professional Conduct demands that nurses put their patients' needs first, nurses must:

- be fully educated in the whole process of transplantation;
- understand their role in transplantation nursing;
- be aware of the ethical issues and principles involved in transplantation;
- be aware of patients' rights;
- educate their patients to an appropriate degree;
- be aware of the influence they have on the decisions that patients make;
- involve themselves in multidisciplinary discussion;
- assertively challenge decisions which they believe are not in the best interests of their patients.

References

Department of Health — NHS Management Executive (1990) *Patient Consent to Examination or Treatment*. HC (90) 22. London, HMSO.

Fletcher, H.R. and Shrigley, R. (1991) Am I entitled to the truth? *Kidney Life*, Summer: 5.

Green, C. (1983) *Organ Transplantation. A Review*. Oxford, The Medicine Publishing Foundation.

Mandell, G.L., Douglas, R.G. and Bennett, J.E. (eds.) (1990) *Principles and Practice of Infectious Diseases* (3rd edn.). Edinburgh, Churchill Livingstone.

UKCC (1992) *Code of Professional Conduct* (3rd edn.). London, UKCC.

United Kingdom Transplant Service (1990) *Transplant Services and Statistics for the United Kingdom and Eire including the UK Transplant Service for 1990 Annual Report* Bristol, UKTS.

United Kingdom Transplant Support Service (1991). Transplant Statistics/January–30 June 1991. *United Kingdom Transplant Support Service Users Bulletin*, **1**:3.

Further Reading

Critical Care Nursing Quarterly (1991) **13**(4).

This issue covers various aspects of transplantation. Of particular relevance are the following articles:

Ethical implications of organ transplantation (pp. 1–7). This article clarifies the ethical issues facing nurses and provides positive guidance.

Renal transplantation: an option for end-stage renal disease patients (pp. 62–71). This article looks at the benefits and the risks of kidney transplantation as well as the psychological effects on patients and their families.

Nursing (1992) **5**(3): 8–16.

This issue contains three articles on accountability. The most relevant, *Breaking the Code*, discusses accountability and the nurse's Code of Conduct.

Nursing Times (1991) **87** (37): 28–31.

The Gift of Life is a short article which describes aspects of organ retrieval, including specific criteria for organ donation and the nurse's role in caring for bereaved relatives.

Whitworth, J.A. and Lawrence, J.R. (eds.) (1987) *Textbook of Renal Disease*. Edinburgh, Churchill Livingstone.

Chapter 20 contains a description of the whole process of kidney transplantation, including the complexities of tissue matching.

Heart and Heart-Lung Transplantation

> He who knows nothing, loves nothing. He who can do
> nothing, understands nothing. He who understands
> nothing is worthless. But he who understands, also loves,
> notices, sees. . . . The more knowledge is inherent in a
> thing, the greater the love. . . . Anyone who imagines that
> all fruits ripen at the same time as strawberries knows
> nothing about grapes.   *Paracelsus*

The first heart transplant in this country was performed
in 1980, the first heart-lung transplant in 1983. Patients
with cystic fibrosis were included in the programme in
1985.

Cardiothoracic transplantation has escalated rapidly in
this country since then. At the time of writing there are
eight designated transplant centres and this number is
likely to increase in the future.

Transplantation is now widely accepted as a possible
option for end stage disease for which no other effective
treatment is available. It is therefore recognised as a life-
saving procedure. The rapid advancement of the programme has been aided by the development of new technology and skills, and the discovery and refinement of
cyclosporin as an immunosuppressant drug. A wide range
of conditions are now considered eligible for transplant,
and the survival rate has improved.

Transplantation is both expensive and labour intensive
and patients must remain immunosuppressed and be followed up for life. Critics argue that the money would be
better spent for the benefit of a greater number on preven-
tive or general medicine.

Transplantation gives rise to both ethical and resource
allocation problems, and poses philosophical questions
about the postponement of fatal disease, the prolonging
of life and the avoidance of death.

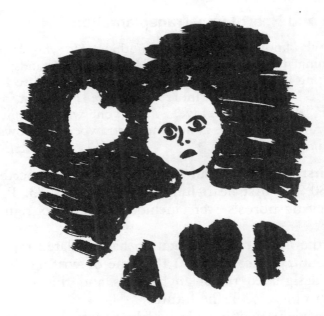

Lack of suitable donor organs significantly limits the programme. Patients are put on a waiting list, categorised according to priority, but many die before a transplant becomes available. Young adults are likely to have a better chance of recovery; do they therefore have more right to the chance of life? What are the other criteria that might make one patient more eligible than another, how tacit or stated are these and whose values do they reflect?

Both selection for transplant and its eventual outcome can seem like a lottery, the prize being life itself, and the cost being borne by many, sometimes including the patient.

This is a question of justice in the sense of fairness of distribution or what is deserved. An injustice occurs when some benefit to which a person is entitled is denied without 'good reason' or when some burden is imposed unduly.

Different transplant centres may establish different criteria for 'good reason', such as age and clinical fitness, although it is widely recognised that poor motivation, failure to comply with treatment and psychiatric or emotional instability are seen as contraindications to transplantation.

This discriminating use of scarce resources may reinforce the idea that some patients are more deserving than others. Society distinguishes between organ failure brought on by congenital defects or other sources beyond control and that brought on by neglect or choice of a dangerous lifestyle. This particular value may seem entirely appropriate, but selection procedures may also less obviously reflect social, racial, sexual and cultural biases institutionalised in society.

Organ donation

The ethics of organ donation are very complex and can only briefly be addressed here.

The Human Organ Transplant Act 1989 prohibits commercial dealings in human organs, places restrictions upon transplants between living persons who are not genetically related and requires certain information to be supplied about transplant operations.

The donor must be certified as brain dead. The Harvard criteria for brain death (Henry and Pashley 1990) are:

- absence of cerebral responsiveness;
- absence of induced or spontaneous movement;
- absence of spontaneous respiration;
- absence of brain stem or deep tendon reflexes.

This definition of death is felt to be unacceptable by some in the medical profession who argue that there are limitations in the brain death criteria, and that those who sign donor cards are unaware of these and the practice of removing organs from a body still supported on external support systems. They maintain that the level of public ignorance in this respect means that donor cards fail to meet the ethical criteria of informed consent, and no attempt is made to redress this.

A nurse working on an intensive care unit may find him or herself caring for a brain stem dead patient who is being artificially kept alive to remain viable as a donor. Caring for a 'living donor' in this way can be very stressful. The patient's dignity must still be respected, and the family's need for consultation and involvement recognised.

Relatives' wishes must always be respected even though the deceased may have carried a donor card. They should not be pressured into agreement to donate an organ or made to feel guilty should they refuse to do so. The only information available to the donor family is the age and sex of the recipient although, if he wishes to, the recipient can contact the donor family through the transplant co-ordinator. The donor's family's need for follow-through and possible counselling should be recognised. The British Organ Donor Society (BODY) aims specifically to identify and respond to the needs of donor families.

Required request

A possible solution to increase the supply of organs is to legislate for **required request**, which would require doctors or nurses to ask relatives of all possible donors whether they agree to organ donation. Special training would be necessary for those involved in this process.

Opting out

In some countries, though not the UK, unless they have specifically stated to the contrary, or their families object, deceased people may automatically become multi-organ donors.

Commercial marketing in organs is seen as ethically objectionable, although the media may promote individual cases in a way that fails to address the uncertainty and complexity of organ donation and transplant procedures. This highlights the critical role played by values concerning justice, truth and respect for the dead.

Process

Transplantation can be broken into distinct phases:

- Assessment.
- Waiting.
- First six months post-transplant.
- Long-term post-transplant.

There are both situational and general ethical considerations encountered by nurses at each stage.

Assessment phase

Patients who agree to a transplant assessment find themselves at the beginning of a long journey which is likely to be very testing and unpredictable, and whose length and destination are by no means certain. An added complication is that the heart is considered the seat of emotion and feeling, that is, the essential source of personality. For example, the husband of a successfully transplanted patient felt unable to send his wife a Valentine card with a heart, because his wife no longer had the heart he had married.

Being told they need a transplant can be a great shock for some patients who may have previously been falsely reassured, or personally denied the severity of their illness. On the other hand, many patients feel relieved that denial need no longer be maintained and they and their family can start dealing with the reality of their illness.

Patients need to be given clear and honest information about the risks of surgery and organ rejection, the possibly long and even fruitless waiting time, and the lifelong need for compliance with treatment. The outcome of the many specific investigations can cause great anxiety and permission must be given for the necessary HIV test.

Assessment includes an appraisal of all the resources available to the patient, including the family who may have to tolerate the high levels of stress implicit in waiting for a life-saving operation and post-surgical care.

Special Considerations

- Patients are sometimes inappropriately assessed for transplant as a way of keeping hope alive and denying mortality. This type of confused thinking might be avoided by asking, what is best for this particular patient? This posits the most basic ethical question, what is happening here?, and any reply must attempt to answer from the patient and carer's point of view. In other words, to do unto others *not* as you would they do unto you, but as they would be done unto.
- Patients should be allowed to refuse assessment without recrimination or implications for their future care. Autonomy means the right to exercise independent choices that may conflict with medical advice. Refusing assessment may be seen as suicidal flight rather than fight and subtle forms of blackmail and pressure used to convince patients to change their minds.
- Informed consent implies that patients *know* what is in their best interests. Levels of expectation and understanding vary widely and information-giving

should be sensitive to the needs of individual patients.

- Helping patients to maintain a positive and constructive attitude towards transplant surgery can conflict with the ethical requirement to discuss the risks of organ rejection and death. Many post-operative patients state that insufficient emphasis was placed on this. A large percentage of patients and their families use denial as a way of coping and will choose to 'hear' only selectively. Respect for patients means acknowledging their defences and what may be their own truth at a given moment in time.
- Patients often need to make an impression of being good and worthy of a transplant. They may feel that their future depends upon the opinions and decisions of others. Subtle forms of bargaining are not uncommon. Patients may become unusually dependent upon those caring for them and/or invest them with unrealistic powers. It is an ethical requirement that nurses need to be aware when this happens and help patients to retain as much autonomy and self-reliance as possible.

Waiting phase

Once accepted and placed on the transplant list, many patients experience feelings of great optimism and a sense of reprieve. After this initial relief, the waiting period can become increasingly anxious and frustrating for the patient and his or her family. Many patients become secretly angry and frightened in their state of limbo and powerlessness. Gradual erosion of optimism is often accompanied by the confusion and complexity of feelings and a sense of personal isolation. Life is perceived to be dependent upon the death of another.

Special considerations

- Drugs such as narcotics and steroids which improve quality of life are reduced or withheld from patients waiting for a transplant. This can increase levels of discomfort and suffering and sometimes mean a protracted, difficult death. It is important to give patients every opportunity to discuss their situation, and for their needs to be acknowledged and validated.
- A time may come when a patient becomes too ill to be eligible for a transplant. The decision to tell a patient that he or she is no longer transplantable seems to be a random and subjective one. A nurse who is aware of a patient's needs may be able to contribute positively to this decision. Despite the obvious benefits of interdisciplinary meetings, organisational structures tend to confine the discussion of issues to segregated groups of various professionals. However, given his or her privileged relationship, a nurse may be required to act as an advocate for the patient — that is, safeguard his or her wellbeing and interest. This may involve conflict with the opinions of others, but is an essential feature in the exercise of accountability.
- Patients may seek false reassurance for unrealistic hopes about the availability and outcome of surgery. Desire to comfort a patient may mean collusion with this denial. Nurses are faced with the need to balance hope for survival against planning for the possibility of death.
- Vulnerability and dependency of patients and the sense of imminence and uncertainty can result in a nurse identifying with the emotions experienced by the patient. It is still important for the patient's own strengths and resources to be acknowledged and to

recognise that many families discover new bonds and loyalties to cope with in this crisis. If the first moral obligation of the helping professions is to be competent, competence in this case always involves a level of self-awareness. This may mean being alert to signals from yourself and others of worry or resentment over the difficulties of reconciling an effective distance with empathy for patients. It is legitimate and necessary to identify the difficulties and seek support in working constructively with them.

The post-transplant phase

However well prepared they were, most patients state that they had not been able to anticipate the full impact of their post-operative experience. This experience is often a mixed one.

During the first few post-operative weeks, patients and their families are often euphoric and emotionally labile. Removal of the immediate threat of death reaffirms the patients' will to live and enhances their capacity to deal with the dual threats of rejection and infection. Patients and their families start feeling less helpless and more in control of their lives once again. The waiting is over and they have joined an exclusive club.

The 'good' patients may now feel that they have to be 'grateful' and may need permission to acknowledge and express negative feelings. They may also experience 'survival guilt' that they have been rescued when others in the same situation have not. The onset of the first rejection episode may bring periods of depression or anger, and a reminder of the vulnerability and dependence on immuno-suppressant therapy.

A number of patients may require extended periods of ventilation, and a small percentage die in the immediate post-operative period. Relatives at least know that the patient made an informed choice to have a transplant and that this opportunity was given.

Special considerations

- Although greatly relieved that the waiting is over, patients may feel overwhelmed by the physical and emotional trauma of transplant surgery and find themselves beset and confused by a quite different set of anxieties.
- Relatives may feel distanced by the technology supporting a patient and the specialist clinical skills of nurses and doctors.
- It is the responsibility of nursing and medical staff that relatives are given clear and understandable information and are involved as much as possible in patient care.
- While expectations have been raised by a transplant and are focused on recovery, it may be difficult to acknowledge that a patient must be allowed to die.
- Decisions regarding the continued use of life support systems should be discussed fully with relatives, and their needs for care and support acknowledged.

The long-term post-transplant phase

Many patients are able to assume relatively normal living patterns and have greatly improved quality of life. However, they are required to adjust their lifestyle and diet and take immunosuppressant drugs for the rest of their lives.

Some experience difficulties in the transition from being a chronically sick and dependent member of a family to becoming reasonably well and self-determining. This change of roles can cause conflict within marriages and

families and may often require the insights and support
of professional counselling.

A number of patients may suffer such severe rejection
episodes that they require a second transplant to survive
and thus must go through the process again. Even so they
may still die.

Many patients, thankful for a second chance, are determined to live their new lives as fully as possible. This
may cause them to deny to themselves and others some
unresolved feelings about the crisis and meaning of transplant surgery, the commitment to after-care and anxiety
for the future.

Special considerations

- Heart and heart-lung transplant is a treatment, not a
  cure, and can present problems at all stages. These
  physical, emotional and spiritual problems may be
  complex and seem to some intractable. It may cause
  some people to question the validity of transplant
  surgery.
- Some patients may require a second transplant and
  the ethics of a patient receiving two sets of organs,
  while others may die for lack of one, may be questioned. Are there times when invasive life-saving
  surgical procedures are excessive and inappropriate
  for a particular patient, and if so, who should contribute to this decision?

James Brown and his son Jonathan suffered from the same
terminal condition. Both had been assessed for a heart
transplant. Jonathan died very suddenly and, shortly
afterwards, his father had a heart transplant. Following post-
operative complications and an extended period of being
ventilated, James Brown underwent a second heart transplant.
This too proved unsuccessful, and following further weeks
being ventilated in intensive care, he died.

It was thought that Mr Brown had not had time to grieve properly for his son, prior to his first transplant, felt guilty that he and not his son had been given this opportunity but felt that he must take it, at least partly for his wife's sake.

Mrs Brown was desperate for her husband to survive and her husband's second transplant was an understandable attempt to thwart a second family death. Nurses and social workers who had known Mr Brown prior to surgery felt that he had neither the resilience nor the motivation to survive a second transplant.

The need not to abandon a patient for whom care has been rendered has to be balanced with the ethical concepts of beneficence (the doing of good) and non-maleficence (doing no harm). Because it is not possible to predict precisely the outcome of surgery, the patient's own truth must be taken into consideration alongside any clinical judgement.

- A small percentage of patients will die of transplant related complications, and all patients will require follow-up and expensive immunosuppressant therapy for the rest of their lives. Thus it may be perceived by some that the net gains of a transplant programme do not justify the considerable and continuous financial outlay, and that justice would be better served if the resources were more effectively used elsewhere.

Summary

Heart and heart-lung transplantation is probably the most dramatic of all transplant surgery. For most lay people it cannot just be perceived as a clinical event, but involves the removal and replacement of the organ most closely associated with someone's personal and emotional identity. The very core of the personality is affected. Myths, fairy tales and history itself testify to the numinous power we attach to this most vital of organs, and we cannot eliminate these associations when discussing transplantation.

Unlike any other kind of transplant surgery, heart transplantation can be seen to offer not just a reprieve, but a symbolic opportunity of a new heart, a metanoia or change of heart, and as such resonates within us something described in most world religions and mythologies, that is, the ability to be transformed and saved. This may well account for some of the mystique which surrounds this particular type of transplant, and the reverence attached to those who perform it. Modern skills and technology have, paradoxically, made manifest ancient beliefs.

Thus it is that heart and heart-lung transplants arouse strong feelings. Understandably, the public image tends to focus on the success stories and it is often only the professionals with long-term involvement who may be aware of the broader picture and the difficulties that may be encountered at every stage.

Nurses may feel ambivalent. On the one hand they may have seen a young patient with cystic fibrosis who through transplantation has been given a whole new lease of life, while on the other hand, they may have seen another patient waiting many months in limbo, only to die a slow and protracted death.

The system may seem random and unpredictable and yet nurses (like their patients) have to tolerate a sense of powerlessness and uncertainty of outcome. This dilemma may be experienced in the balance required in helping to prepare patients and their families realistically for what may be ahead, while at the same time helping them to remain positive and hopeful.

Most people cannot remain purposefully engaged in a situation of human conflict or suffering, unless they feel that they have something positive and effective to contribute. It may be helpful for nurses to have made their own 'overall' decision about the ethical values of this type of transplant, that *it is* or that *it is not* a morally and practically justifiable procedure. If a nurse feels it is not, it may be better not to work with such patients. The 1989 UKCC Advisory Document *Exercising Accountability* states that since the law provides no basic right to such refusal, it is imperative that practitioners should be careful not to accept employment in a post where it is known that a form of treatment to which they have a conscientious objection is regularly used.

If a nurse feels that transplantation is morally justified, that nurse may choose to work with transplant patients but be aware of the compromises and conflicts encountered and, where necessary, act as the patient's advocate.

Patients have very different ways of dealing with threat; some may be able to acknowledge risk and fear, others need to deny it. Patients being assessed and waiting for a transplant are uniquely vulnerable. A patient, while waiting for a transplant, wrote movingly of his predicament and needs in two newspaper articles. He wrote of the totally abnormal predicament he found himself in and commented that sympathy was used as a substitute for comprehension and expressed in ways which, although unquestionably well intentioned, tended to be patronising.

Nurses involved in the total care of their patients need to take on board the wide range of hopes and fears, the sense of fatalism and uncertainty, and the bizarre balance of waiting for a death to give life.

Even the most rational person cannot always equate the conflicts inherent in the situation, for they touch on deep-seated taboos within ourselves and can only assume some coherence through an understanding of our own values, a sense of what is right and wrong and the importance we attach to life and death. It is our own personal ethics as well as those which inform our professional standards which will help us retain a sense of meaning and integrity.

The considerable financial resources put into the transplant programme finally benefit a relatively small number of people, and no human audit is taken of those who were not eligible for assessment, those who failed to meet the assessment criteria, those who died while waiting and those for whom transplant was unsuccessful.

However, there is wide acceptance that the heart and heart-lung transplant programme continues to offer hope for many who would otherwise have none, and a greatly enhanced quality of life for those who have been successfully transplanted.

Philosophically and theologically, it might be seen that we are all part of a corporate being, members one of another, and fundamental to humanity is our dependence rather than independence. In this sense, organ donation can be a gratefully accepted gift.

This does not refute the fact that organ donation and transplantation pose conflicting ethical demands and might be indefensible if justice were to be based on the concept of the greatest good for the greatest number. In working with transplant patients, we are required to address the most fundamental human questions for which, quite properly, there are no simple and clear cut answers.

The ethical principles of justice, beneficence, consent and truth which should inform all medical practice can perhaps only in the end, be realised in the skill, empathy and service of practitioners able to interpret and advocate for what a patient's own truth may be. Over two thousand years ago Paracelsus understood that respect and attention to the individual were the only real criteria, and all contemporary knowledge gained since then will never allow grapes to ripen like strawberries.

References

Henry C. and Pashley, G. (1990) *Health Ethics*. Lancaster, Quay
   Publishing.
UKCC (1989) *Exercising Accountability*. London, UKCC.

Further Reading

Beer, S. (1990) New lease of life. *Nursing Times*, **86**, 29 July:
   34–7.
Caplin, A.L. (1987) Equity in the selection and recipients for
   cardiac transplants. *Transplantation of the Heart*, **75**(1): 10–19.
Christopherson, L.K. (1987) Cardiac transplantation — a
   psychological perspective. *Transplantation of the Heart*, **75**(1):
   1–10.
Gould, D. (1986) Death's sting, society tomorrow. *The Times*,
   August 6th.
*Guidance on the Requirements of The Human Organ Transplants
   Act 1989* (1990) London, HMSO.
Iwerson, E. (1988) Life at what cost? *American Journal of Nurs-
   ing*, May: 639.
Kuhn, W.F., Myers, B., Brennan, A.F., Davis, M.H.,
   Lippmann, S.B., Gray, L.A. and Pool, G.E. (1988) Psycho-
   pathology in heart and transplant patients. *The Journal of
   Heart Transplantation*, **7**(3): 223–5.
Marsden, C. (1985) Ethical issues in a heart transplant pro-
   gramme. *Heart and Lung*, **5**, September: 495–8.
The National Commission for the Protection of Human Sub-
   jects of Biomedic and Behavioural Research (1979) The
   Belmont Report. London, HMSO.
Roach, M.S. (1986) Reflections on the ethics of organ donation
   and retrieval. *Halifax Herald*, July 25.
Roche, E. (1987) Ethical decisions in nursing. *Professional Nurse*,
   March: 164–6.
UKCC (1992) *Code of Professional Conduct* (3rd edn.). London,
   UKCC.
UKCC (1989) *Exercising Accountability* London, UKCC.
Wainwright, E. and Lum, L.C. (1986) The ethics of cardiac
   transplantation. *British Journal of Hospital Medicine*, July: 68–9.

Useful address

BODY – The British Organ Donor Society
Balsham
Cambridge CB1 6DL
Telephone: (0223) 893636

Other Transplants

This chapter would not be complete without at least mentioning some of the other organ transplant possibilities available.

The most common and the most successful type of organ transplant is of skin, closely followed by corneal grafts.

A type of transplant which has been much discussed since its first use is that of fetal brain cell transplant for patients suffering from Parkinson's disease. The link with abortion has made discussion much more complicated. The Polkinghorne Committee (1989), which reported on this practice, stressed the need to ensure 'a separation of the supply of fetal tissue from its use.'

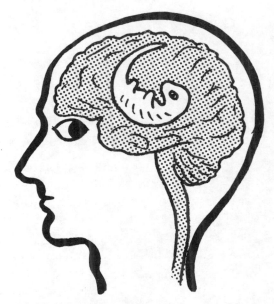

Easton and Lamb (1991) point out that the quantity of fetal cells used for any one transplant in no way justifies the fear that women might be encouraged to have an abortion for possible transplant purposes — and that this could be financially exploited. But at the same time they suggest that over 110 000 people suffer from Parkinson's disease in the UK who could all, potentially at least, benefit from a transplant.

In its series of cards on *Issues in Nursing and Health*, the Royal College of Nursing (RCN) has produced *Fetal Cell Transplantation Guidance for Nurses*. This recommends that nurses involved directly or indirectly should:

- familiarise themselves with the Code of Practice in the Polkinghorne Report;
- satisfy themselves as far as possible that the Code is being adhered to;
- give support and assistance to the woman, not only in relation to her decision about the termination of pregnancy but also subsequently in relation to consent to the use of fetal tissue for research or therapeutic purposes;
- provide the best standard of nursing care, including psychological care, before and after termination of pregnancy;
- provide the best standard of nursing care for the recipient of the transplant material.

At a conference of the Society of Neurosciences in Toronto, in 1988, 'US and Swedish scientists spoke positively of an alternative course for patients suffering from Alzheimer's and Parkinson's disease. This rival therapy involves genetically altering the tissues taken from the patient, probably skin cells, and grafting them to parts of the brain, thus avoiding the need for donor tissue' (Easton and Lamb 1991). If this research becomes practice, the ethical problems posed by fetal cell transplants for Parkinson's disease may become irrelevant. However, other research may use similar material for other diseases and conditions in the future. The issue may not be solved by hoping that it will disappear, but only by being addressed.

The possibility of xenografts, ie transplantation of organs from different species, is another issue which will need to be addressed sooner or later. Already, in 1990 in the USA, one person has received the heart of a baboon, and research in this field is continuing.

The issues which concern nurses who care for patients waiting to receive organ transplants seem to centre particularly around the position of nurses within the caring team. That position does not appear always to be one of equality with doctors when it concerns the contribution nurses make to decisions to be taken. Holistic care is only holistic when all the lines of communication are functioning openly.

Issues of advocacy and informed consent are particularly relevant in this area, but aspects of accountability, particularly moral accountability, also figure. The nursing care given can only be accountable when it is honest, enhances care in the fullest sense, and empowers nurses to be fully functioning persons and professionals.

Practices at the frontiers of the acceptable always pose ethical problems, yet care only advances with possibilities being available, being used, being refined and challenging views and values about caring.

References

Easton, S. and Lamb, D. (1991) Transplanting Fetal Tissue. *Nursing Times*, **87**(31): 39–40.
Polkinghorne Committee (1989) *Review of the Guidance on the Research Use of Fetuses and Fetal Material*. London, HMSO.
Royal College of Nursing (1991) *Fetal Cell Transplantation Guidance for Nurses*. London, RCN.

CHAPTER 3

Cardio-pulmonary Resuscitation

Paul Cain

Cardio-pulmonary resuscitation (CPR) is a procedure which
every nurse learns early on. But is the procedure right for
every patient, and if not, when is and when isn't it appropriate?
   The many ways in which CPR is questioned and debated are
detailed in this chapter. The reasons for judging are outlined,
and guidance on decision-making is given, based on practical,
philosophical and ethical considerations.

If you are a practising nurse of some years' experience (or
even of very little), you may well have been involved in
resuscitation attempts, and experienced the demands on
your emotional resources that these can make. You are
also likely to have cared for patients for whom a 'Do not
resuscitate' order had been given. In either case, you may
have experienced moral perplexity, even though the
decision to resuscitate, or not to resuscitate, was probably
not yours.

Perhaps the key moral question for you was, is it right
that this patient should be resuscitated? Or maybe you felt
that a decision not to resuscitate a patient was mistaken.
Perhaps your question was, shouldn't this patient have
been consulted first? Or the relatives? Or maybe you were
uncertain what was expected of you, because there was a
lack of clear instructions or guidelines. Perhaps there were
clear instructions and you felt that, morally, in this situation, you ought not to follow them. Maybe you felt that
your views could and should have been sought.

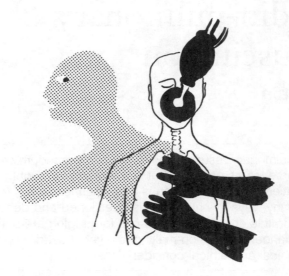

Certainly it is the case that since its inception as a life-saving procedure in 1960, CPR, as cardio-pulmonary resuscitation has come to be termed, has been a focus of professional and ethical concern. It may be useful to illustrate this.

As early as 1966, a survey by the RCN Ward and Departmental Section, promoted in part by nurses' dilemmas over who should be resuscitated, elicited comments of relief that 'something is being done about the problem'. A report of the survey (*Nursing Times* 1966) referred to 'nurses' concern about their responsibility in resuscitating patients suffering from cardiac arrest'. The report noted that 'their concern is not only in defining their responsibility, it is for the patients and their relatives and for the young and inexperienced student or pupil nurses who may have to make a life and death decision without the necessary experience or guidance to influence that decision.'

One of the aims of the survey was to discover how

many hospitals (there were 152 surveyed) had policies that could guide decision-making: more than half said they had no policy.

In 1977, a research study (Gaskell) involving 103 nurses in three hospitals found that a majority of the nurses (88 per cent) sometimes had to decide for themselves whether or not to initiate resuscitation. For the most part, instructions were lacking: 54 nurses were only 'occasionally' told in advance whom or whom not to resuscitate.

A continuing lack of policy, relating in this case to how resuscitation decisions should be reached and communicated within the health care team, was highlighted in a complaint to the Health Service Commissioner in 1990. A woman was given a 'Do not resuscitate' order, but recovered and was discharged from hospital; the existence of the order became known to her son who had not been consulted. The Commissioner commented on a 'worrying divergence of policy on consulting relatives'. In this case, the consultant believed their attitude should be taken into account in arriving at a decision, whereas the junior medical staff did not think this was required or even appropriate. There was at that time no agreed policy.

Even if you have not been directly involved in resuscitation attempts yourself, you may nevertheless be aware through accounts in the nursing journals of how ethically problematic they can be. Over a long period they have frequently carried articles reflecting the moral worry that CPR can provoke.

For example, an article in the *Nursing Times* (Canham and Gunga 1985) referred to the 'discomfiture' most experienced nurses feel at the 'widespread and indiscriminate use of CPR'. This article brought to the fore the way in which situations involving decisions about resuscitation may confront a junior nurse. The authors write, 'Doctors and experienced nurses . . . are rarely present when a patient's life comes to an unexpected end. They escape the torment of deciding whether to confer a peaceful demise or the dramatic mobilisation of hospital forces upon a lifeless body. The person at that bedside may be only 19 and no-one will be there to tell her with absolute authority what action she should take'.

An article in *Nursing* (Dolan 1988) quotes two cases from a hospital where there *was* a clear policy, that of resuscitating everyone regardless. One nurse was haunted by the memory of having to attempt resuscitation on a patient with infectious hepatitis and AIDS. She said, 'it was terrible. With every compression, blood flowed from his mouth, so giving him oxygen was nearly impossible . . . Wasn't our futile attempt to save his life unfair to him and to us?' Another nurse spoke of doing CPR on a patient riddled with bone cancer: 'I could feel the crunch of broken bone on each compression. What was I doing?'.

And yet, where a nurse exercises her own judgement, in order, in her view, to promote the interests of a patient, this may be professionally risky. The *Nursing Times* (1983) carried a report of a nurse who chose to let an elderly man die rather than call an emergency resuscitation team. She was dismissed on grounds of gross misconduct. At the industrial tribunal considering her appeal against unfair dismissal, a hospital registrar said she had no right to decide whether or not a patient should be resuscitated. The nurse told the tribunal, 'I thought I would let him die peacefully. In my mind he was already dead'.

These references indicate the concern that the practice of cardio-pulmonary resuscitation has provoked. In 1990, it was one of the areas raised by practitioners to be addressed by the UKCC Standards and Ethics Committee. This concern is also reflected in the RCN's current discussions to develop guidelines specifically relating to resuscitation. It is, of course, also reflected in this chapter.

The questions we need to address are also indicated.

They are the following: What would be morally acceptable grounds for decisions not to resuscitate a patient?
Who should take these decisions? What in particular
should be the role of the nurse? And to what extent should
there be guidelines to shape decision-making and the communication of decisions within the health care team?

These questions provide a framework for this chapter,
the initial question being, what would be morally acceptable grounds for decisions not to resuscitate a patient?
Firstly, though, we should consider a view which implies
that no reason is *good enough* to justify decisions not to
resuscitate.

No reasons are good enough to justify 'Do Not Resuscitate' orders

Some would hold that cardio-pulmonary resuscitation
should be denied to no-one. This view follows from a
particular understanding of the 'sanctity of life' principle,
according to which life is of intrinsic value, respecting
life is of overriding importance, and so withholding a
necessary means of averting death is morally unacceptable. J David Bleich (1989), a Jewish rabbi, expresses this
view clearly:

> Not only is life in general of infinite and inestimable value,
> but every moment of life is of inestimable value as well.
> The quality of life which is preserved is thus never a factor
> to be taken into consideration. Neither is the length of the
> patient's life expectancy a controlling factor.

Consistent with this, he claims that the physician's duty
is to work for:

> not simply . . . the restoration of health, but . . . the
> restoration of even a single moment of life.

This form of the sanctity of life principle clearly supports a prohibition of abortion, and of any form of euthanasia; it also appears to prohibit any withholding of treatment that might prolong life, so 'Do not resuscitate' orders are out.

If as a nurse you held this view, you would be open to the most agonising dilemmas, since your belief would commit you to do all you could to resuscitate a patient, even though a doctor had placed a 'Do not resuscitate' instruction in the patient's medical notes. Is there any way in which the values of the sanctity of life and respect for life can be retained without this radical implication?

A perspective which retains these notions without this implication must draw a distinction between life as an organic metabolic process and human life. From this perspective, life in the first sense has instrumental value: it is a necessary means to the possibility of human life. Distinctively human life has intrinsic value because of its particular potentialities and capacities, for example the potential and capacity to form relationships, to exercise choice, to be happy. So, in this view, the overriding source of value and object of respect is personal life, or the life of persons.

The implications of this perspective for using, or withholding, CPR are clear. Where those qualities and capacities that constitute the value of personal life are absent, or are seriously eroded, for example by chronic illness, then there is a case for withholding CPR. Withholding CPR would, therefore, other things being equal, not conflict with a sense of the value of life and respect for life: it might very well be an expression of value and respect. In particular, if a patient expressed a clear wish not to be resuscitated, respect for life can be expressed by respecting that wish; and even where a clear wish not to be resuscitated has not been expressed, it might be that to administer CPR would violate the duty of respect. For example, where patients are in the last stages of a terminal illness, resuscitation may rob dying of any dignity, subjecting the patient to both the trauma of resuscitation and the technological trappings of subsequent intensive care.

So the principle of respect for life, and a conviction of the value of life, does not necessarily imply resuscitation at all costs. It depends on how 'life' is understood, and on what its value is taken to consist of. This dilemma is the fundamental ethical problem related to CPR. If the second perspective is adopted, other ethical issues are raised of 'good reasons' for decisions not to resuscitate. We will now consider them.

What are morally acceptable grounds for decisions not to resuscitate?

Some of the reasons that are commonly cited are the age of the patient, the patient's quality of life, the patient's condition and the patient's wishes. In each case one may want to ask: is this a good reason and is it a sufficient reason?

1. Age as a reason

Many people think that age provides a good, ie a morally justifying, reason for withholding resuscitation. Indeed, you may think so yourself, since one piece of research (Stewart and Rai 1985), surveying nurses' attitudes to resuscitation, found that 82.5 per cent of those questioned felt that a patient's advanced age 'should be a very important or quite important factor'. In another piece of research (Candy 1991) it was found that 'all patients on geriatric wards were "not for resuscitation" even though some may have been as young as 60 years, and many were subsequently discharged'.

One reason for thinking that age *is* morally relevant to decisions not to resuscitate is that it may make a good outcome of resuscitation attempts unlikely. However, this does not appear with any certainty to be the case. In a review of research on this question, it has been noted that 'most studies have failed to confirm that age has an independent influence on the prognosis for survival after resuscitation . . .' (Bayer et al 1985) and that '. . . an inadequate number of otherwise healthy elderly patients has been studied to determine whether or not age contributes entirely independently to the prognosis' (Murphy et al 1989).

Another reason for thinking that age is morally relevant is the belief that old people would not want to be resuscitated. It may be true of an individual person that old age is a reason for their not wishing to be resuscitated: in individual cases it may be morally relevant. But is it true of the elderly and the old as a category? If it were, this would provide some justification for debarring people from receiving CPR on the basis of age. You may feel intuitively that this is unlikely to be true: after all, people differ. If so, your feeling is backed up by research. For example, although one piece of research (Fusgen and Summar 1978), following up 18 survivors of CPR, half of whom were under and half over the age of 60, found that none of the over–60s would agree to be resuscitated if need be. Other research (Gunasekera et al 1986), surveying opinion among 134 elderly patients, found that 89.6 per cent of patients felt that resuscitation should not be withheld from the elderly. Yet other research (Bayer et al 1985) found that none of 13 elderly patients who had been successfully resuscitated expressed regrets.

Another reason for thinking age should be a factor in resuscitation decisions is a version of the 'good innings' argument. Old people, it might be claimed, have had their 'innings', and since there are limited resources, it is only fair that these should go to younger people, who have their life ahead of them.

What are we to make of this argument? In the first place, it is clear that resuscitation does use up substantial resources for, if successful, patients invariably spend time in intensive care. Secondly, it is clearly true that resources are limited, and some way has to be found of discriminating between categories of patients, and categories of care: prioritisation is unavoidable. It is also true that there is a precedent for an age-based standard in the area of heart transplants: people over 60 do not qualify. But *is* age a fair basis for discrimination (rather than, say, need)? The practice of giving people unfavourable treatment on the basis of age alone is what is meant by 'ageism' and would be widely condemned, so is there a reason for supposing that an age-based standard can apply fairly here, that in some way resuscitation is morally different? Can an age-based standard avoid the charge of being simply arbitrary?

A case might be made from a Utilitarian standpoint. From this standpoint the overriding concern is to maximise welfare, and it could be argued that welfare would be maximised if an age-based rule were applied. How would the argument go? It would have to be claimed that younger people, as a rule, have greater social utility, are, for example, more likely to be in employment, or to be bringing up children. Younger people, it would be argued, therefore contribute more to society, and so to the general welfare.

You may feel that this is a persuasive point of view. On the other hand, a counter-argument could claim that 'social utility' is not just a matter of making an economic contribution, or bringing up children. For example, old people make an invaluable contribution as grandparents. And might not a society which made every effort to value old people be happier (have more 'welfare') than one which systematically denied them access to particular benefits?

The difficulty, here, is in weighing up and quantifying the consequences for welfare of having an age-based standard, and then comparing those with the consequences of having some other standard which does not discriminate against people on the basis of age. And, as we have seen, another difficulty is that we might not agree about what values should go into the calculation.

The Utilitarian perspective does at least rescue the age-based standard from a charge of arbitrariness: it gives it a rationale. But does it rescue it from the charge of being unfair? If fairness is simply a matter of applying the same rules (whatever they are) equally to all, then it is fair. But clearly this view will not do: it would, for example, sanction the strict application of racist policies. Fairness has, also, to be a matter of what the rules are, and whether they discriminate on morally acceptable grounds between individuals and groups.

Perhaps, in the end, age, whether or not morally acceptable as a reason for 'Do not resuscitate' orders, is not a necessary consideration. The assumption was that given limited resources, some prioritisation must be made, but maybe other factors, such as patients' wishes, the condition of patients, or their quality of life, will be an entirely effective way of ensuring a suitable distribution of resources.

2. Quality of life as a reason

As a nurse, you have probably worked with patients whose quality of life was so poor that you felt that any attempt to resuscitate them, should occasion arise, would be unjustifiable. Perhaps they had very limited capacities, or were in constant pain; or their condition was such that, should they survive any resuscitation attempt, they would have to face years of painful operations. (This may be the case, for example, with spina bifida babies.) Perhaps you knew that resuscitation, if successful, would be likely to be followed by a period in intensive care, with its additional demands. For these patients, you may have felt, death would be a merciful release.

'Quality of life' as a reason for withholding resuscitation attempts certainly does seem more obviously acceptable and less morally contentious, than age. It can be thought of as expressing what is implied in two of the principles many would hold to be important in health care: beneficence, that is, the obligation to promote welfare, and non-maleficence, the obligation not to cause unnecessary harm. If quality of life were very poor, to take active steps to prolong that life might be felt to violate these principles.

There is, however, a worry about this criterion, for many features of life combine to make up its quality, which features are morally relevant to a decision to withhold resuscitation? Research (Farber et al 1985) has shown that CPR decisions may be influenced by whether the patient lacks support systems (eg he or she is a 'street person', or is mentally retarded or institutionalised). Such judgements clearly move way outside medical expertise, and appear to involve evaluations of what kinds of life have value and are worth attempting to prolong.

The worry of being on a 'slippery slope' here underlies the reservation some writers have expressed about 'quality of life' judgements. Kass (1980), for example, writes that:

> such a move also invites considerations of 'social worthiness' or other alien matters to contaminate medical decisions, with not only individual lives, but our very reverence for life, in jeopardy. The consideration in medicine of quality of life, it is correctly said, was the fundamental error of the Nazi physicians.

Is it possible to resist a slide down the slippery slope and yet to retain quality of life criteria?

Perhaps you will agree that what is essential in resisting this slide is that we should try to see things from the patient's point of view. The patient's life may lack many of the features that anyone would agree are objectively important and desirable, for example mobility or freedom from pain, but they may still experience their life as valuable to them. So the patient's wishes must be all-important in 'quality of life' decisions.

Of course, where it is hard, or impossible, to gain access to what the patient wants (perhaps he or she is senile, comatose or profoundly mentally retarded), decisions by the health care team, in conjunction with the patient's relatives, in terms of some objective marks of what counts as acceptable quality, may have to be made. These decisions will at times be open to question since, although there may be agreement on what are relevant criteria (for example, level of pain, capacity for enjoyment or ability to relate to others), there will always be scope for disagreement about what weight should be accorded to these criteria in particular cases: what level of incapacity is acceptable? how much pain? what degree of ability to relate to others?

As earlier stated 'the patient's wishes must be all-important in "quality of life" decisions'. Since, as discussed below, it may be difficult to find out what the patient wants (indeed even the patient may be unsure) this places a particular responsibility on the health care team to develop the kind of relationship with the patient that enables the expression (and identification) of the patient's true wishes. Also, where a patient fails to value his or her life, the importance of the care expressed by the health care team is evident, since the capacity to value one's own life is shaped so much by how much we feel ourselves to be valued by others.

3. The patient's condition as a reason

'Condition' refers primarily to category of disease, and secondarily to whether the disease is in its early stages or advanced, whether there is hope of a cure or not. Different diseases give rise to different prognoses, and for some the prognosis of a good recovery after resuscitation is minimal.

In a review of the research literature, Blackhall (1987) noted that 'survival after CPR is related to the underlying illness that leads to the arrest, and that patients with certain conditions very rarely survive'. This claim can be supported by reference to some of these research findings.

In a study (Bedell and Delbanco 1984) of 294 patients who had had a cardiac arrest and CPR, it was found that no patient with metastatic cancer survived until discharge, nor did any patient with an acute stroke, sepsis or anaemia. Only 3 per cent of patients with renal failure survived. In a study of 1063 patients over a 10-year period, it was found that no patients with cancer or gastrointestinal haemorrhage survived (Peatfield et al 1977). In another study of 552 patients (Johnson et al 1967) no patient with sepsis, cancer or gastrointestinal haemorrhage survived until discharge from hospital. Another study (Murphy et al 1989) reported that only one patient, out of 237 surveyed, survived out of those with asystole, electromechanical dissociation or agonal rhythms. The authors of the study concluded that 'certain trends in our data help to profile the patient for whom cardiopulmonary resuscitation is futile. Patients with significant impairment (acute or chronic) in almost any organ system . . . have poor prognoses'. These references bear out the claim that 'survival after CPR is related to the underlying illness'.

Given the invasiveness of CPR, the threat to dignity,

and the risks involved of part survival in a deeply damaged, possibly vegetative state, it must, therefore, be the
case that the patient's condition may be a good reason, a
morally relevant reason, for 'Do not resuscitate' decisions.
The moral equation, in which possible harms are balanced
against possible benefits, may tell against attempts to
resuscitate.

There are, however, two points to be made. Firstly, it
is the prognosis of the condition that is the relevant point.
This is worth emphasising in view of research (Wachter
et al 1989) which found that physicians tended to give
'Do not resuscitate' orders much more frequently to
patients with AIDS or lung cancer than to those with
cirrhosis and varices or congestive heart failure with cor-
onary artery disease *in spite of the fact that reviews of the
literature indicate that all these diseases have similar prognoses.*
The possibility of subjective bias in relation to disease
categories must, therefore, be held in check by reference
to the prognosis.

Secondly, the fact that 'patients with certain conditions
very rarely survive' implies that patients with those conditions do sometimes survive; hence we have to ask, is
condition and prognosis a sufficient reason for 'Do not
resuscitate' orders? Is there not moral space for the claim
that, even where there is much risk and a poor prognosis,
a patient's wishes should in principle have overriding
authority? This point is discussed next.

4. The patient's wishes as a reason

Whether or not the patient's wishes should override 'Do
not resuscitate' decisions, you may agree that the
patient's wishes must be held to constitute a good reason
for decisions not to resuscitate. The sense in which this
is so can be seen in relation to the principle of autonomy,
for to impose treatment on a patient who competently

rejects it is clearly a failure to respect the patient's autonomy.

If the patient's wishes are a morally relevant reason, finding out what she or he wishes is a moral imperative. What are the problems and possibilities here?

Research shows that patients' wishes are not always sought. For example, research by Candy (1991) found that in one hospital patients over 60 were routinely, ie presumably without consultation, given 'Do not resuscitate' orders. Candy learned from her informants (71 student nurses from two district general hospitals) that 'neither patients nor relatives were involved in the decision about whether or not to resuscitate'. Bedell and Delbanco (1984) found that out of 151 physicians, only 15 who believed in discussing resuscitation with patients actually talked with these patients before the arrest. Evans and Brody (1985), in research carried out at three teaching hospitals, found that 'for the vast majority of patients who were to be resuscitated, that decision was made without either patient or family input'.

So, patients' wishes are not always sought. It is not hard to suggest reasons why this is so. There may be difficulties of communication, whether emotional (the patient may be anxious or depressed), or mechanical (he or she may be intubated). The patient may be a neonate, a young child or mentally impaired. Above all, difficulties may arise from the nature of what is to be communicated. Nolan (1987) draws attention to the fact that resuscitation and its withholding can have 'multiple and sometimes conflicting meanings for patients, families and clinicians'; she notes the risks that attempts at resuscitation can carry risks 'of the most fearful aspects of impending death: pain, isolation, violence, and loss of control', a balancing of the certainty of death if resuscitation is not attempted against the risk of a process of dying that is 'lonely, mechanical and dehumanised' (Kübler-Ross 1969). No wonder then that many clinicians shrink from the task of educating the patient thoroughly in the nature of the procedures involved.

We might then, with reason, intuitively suppose that the process of seeking the patient's wishes about CPR would be distressing. That this may be so is borne out by Schade and Muslin's (1989) discussion of seven cases, where discussion of resuscitation with the patient did take place, with unhappy consequences. What they judge to have been the effect on patients includes 'psychological discomfort and disarray', 'anguish', depression and fright.

In view of this you may feel that, although in principle a patient's wishes should count, in practice they should not be directly sought: we should rely on empathetic guesswork, or the views of relatives. You may feel that here the principles of beneficence (the duty to promote welfare) and non-maleficence (the duty not to cause unnecessary harm) outweigh autonomy. In particular, your experience may be that patients often do not wish to be autonomous, their illness bringing with it a desire to relinquish the burdens of decision-making and welcome for an authoritarian figure (the doctor) who decides on their behalf.

Perhaps, though, it is too easy to conclude that as a rule patients' wishes should not be directly sought — 'easy' since no doubt such discussions as are envisaged make emotional demands on the doctor or nurse as well. The fact that discussions about resuscitation may be upsetting does not entail that such discussions should not take place: it *may* imply that in particular cases discussion should not be taken very far; it *might* justify in particular cases a decision not to engage in discussing the issue at all; but, given the importance of autonomy as a value, all that is implied *as a general rule* is that the way in which such discussions are initiated and carried through is all-important. (Schade and Muslin, who, as we saw, high-lighted the potential distress such discussions may cause, propose a 'careful and cautious delivery of information, guided by patient feedback'.)

The fact that discussions about resuscitation may be upsetting underlines, again, the importance of the relationship between physician and patient and between nurse and patient, if only so that judgements about what a patient can cope with psychologically can be accurately made. It also underlines the importance of communication between medical and nursing staff so that knowledge of the patient as a person (his or her emotional and mental state, character and personality, as well as physical con-dition) can be shared, and damaging errors of judgement avoided.

In the development of this relationship the importance of time and the absence of pressure are arguably essential. This point has been made by O'Neill (1984):

> Given some capacities for autonomous action, whatever
> can be made comprehensible and refusable by patients can
> be treated as subject to their consent — or refusal. This
> may require doctors and others to avoid haste and
> pressure, to counteract the intimidation of unfamiliar,
> technically bewildering and socially alien medical
> environments. Without such care in imparting information
> and proposing treatment, the consent patients give to their
> treatment will lack the autonomous character which would
> show that they have not been treated paternally but rather
> as persons.

All of the above underlines the importance of the nurse's role, for it will be he or she who has the most intimate and consistent contact with the patient. It points to an ethical obligation on those who are responsible for

allocating resources to ensure that the nurse–patient
ratio is sufficiently favourable to allow for such personal,
time-consuming relationships, and to an obligation on
nurses and doctors to collaborate, as advocates for their
patients, in bringing this aspect of patient care to the
attention of those who hold the purse-strings.

Who Should Decide?

Normally, decisions about resuscitation are taken by
medical staff. As one nurse commented: 'It's usually up
to the consultant or registrar in my experience'. It is worth
considering the possible justifications for this. They are
of two kinds: an appeal to expertise, and an appeal to
accountability.

The appeal to expertise presupposes that resuscitation
decisions are exclusively, or at least primarily, matters of
expertise, but this is clearly not the case. Expertise relates
to matters of fact, and implies the ability to identify the
facts and predict outcomes. Thus medical expertise
involves diagnosis and prognosis. However, the move
from claims about what is the case (the medical facts, the
diagnosis) and what will be the case (the prognosis) to
what ought to be done involves a value judgement, for
example a value judgement that the risk of CPR is not
worth taking (the chances of survival are too slim), or that
the quality of life that may be hoped for is too reduced, or
that the length of predicted survival is too short (the illness
is 'terminal'), and so on. Such judgements are clearly
moral value judgements, for they relate to what constitutes the weal or woe, the fundamental interests and welfare of particular people.

It follows from this that if the only consideration is the
kind of decision involved, doctors are not self-evidently

those who should decide: they are not, by virtue of their training, moral experts (indeed it is not clear of what moral expertise would consist).

This line of argument does not, of course, lead to the conclusion that doctors should not decide. Many medical decisions have a moral dimension: medicine has never been merely a matter of technical expertise: it has always been conceived of as a profession involving moral agency. Hence it is open to us to consider the second ground of appeal.

The appeal to accountability is more secure, for while all members of the health care team carry responsibilities in relation to patient care according to their particular role, and are accountable for these, the overall responsibility, and so accountability, lies with the doctor. Therefore, it may be argued, both the burden and the right to take decisions about resuscitation lie with the doctor.

It could be suggested though, that there is one clear limit on this right, ie, where the patient is competent, and expresses a clear wish not to be resuscitated. Where the wish that has been expressed clearly represents the patient's viewpoint, it would be morally wrong to decide otherwise. To say that in such circumstances the patient's wishes should be decisive is equivalent to saying that the patient should decide. The doctor's responsibility, and that of the health care team, is to ascertain what it is that the patient wants.

I think it is less clear that the decision to be resuscitated, should need arise, must in all cases, including those where the doctor judges resuscitation to be futile, rest with the patient. What is at issue is the doctor's right to refuse treatment that he or she holds to be futile, or in some other way inappropriate. Is there this right of decision?

What process of decision-making is ethically indicated?

The foregoing discussion, in which arguments supporting the doctor's right of decision were considered, did not address the question of how decisions should be reached. In now raising the question of the process of decision-making, I have in mind the thought that the process itself may have implications for the welfare both of patients and staff. Any process which tends to minimise the emotional and moral costs of resuscitation can be said to be 'ethically indicated'.

There are various possibilities, of which I shall discuss three: an appeal to rules; the exercise of individual judgement; collaborative discussion.

Appeal to rules?

The value of having rules is that they can provide clear indications as to how to act in particular situations, laying down what would be the right or wrong thing to do. The drawback of having rules is that if rigidly adhered to, they can lead to abuse. Certainly this is the case in relation to decisions about resuscitation.

An example of an abusive situation arising as a result of the application of strict rules is reported by Karen Ellis, (1987) who at the time was a staff nurse in the intensive care unit at Williamsburg Community Hospital, USA. Here the rule was, no DNR order without the family's permission. In this case the patient was 76 years old, he had been in the ICU for two months and was dependent on a mechanical ventilator. He was on haemodialysis because of kidney failure. He suffered from an antibiotic-resistant infection, as a result of which his tracheostomy site leaked green pus. He had pressure sores. He had become a skeleton. He was in a coma, and his only response was to make a grimace when he was suctioned. Karen was on duty the night that his condition began to deteriorate further, his cardiac monitor alarm sounded, his heart rate slowed, then stopped altogether. Because there was no DNR order, the nurse felt obliged to start CPR. She says that when the doctor arrived she asked him angrily '. . . why didn't you write out a DNR order?'. The answer was '. . . I couldn't do that without the consent of his family'. It appears that the sister, his only relative, had refused to listen to any suggestion that her brother should be allowed to die peacefully.

Here was a situation where practice in relation to a particular patient was bound by a rule, in the case of the physician by the rule that there should be no DNR orders without the family's permission, in the case of the nurse by the rule that CPR must be initiated except where DNR orders had been recorded. Since it appears to be the case that what resulted was deeply abusive, it is arguable that rules that are given absolute status, that are allowed to over-ride individual judgement, are not appropriate.

Another attempt to apply rules was a memorandum issued by the physician superintendent of Neasden hospital in 1967 to all medical officers and senior nursing staff, which laid down that 'The following patients are not to be resuscitated: very elderly, over 65 years; malignant disease; chronic chest disease; chronic renal disease'.

This rule runs the risk of leading to abuse of patients by excluding such morally relevant factors as quality of life, and the wishes of the patient, in addition to introducing a morally problematic criterion of age. (The relevance of the individual case, and individual judgement was acknowledged by the Ministry of Health which issued a statement about this memorandum following a public outcry, to the effect that 'no patient should be excluded from consideration for resuscitation by reason of age or diagnostic classification alone, and without regard to all individual circumstances'.)

Could it not be argued that the rule 'the patient's wishes should in all circumstances be respected' can be applied without risk of abuse? Isn't this, of all rules, the one which can and should apply?

Is it, however, certain that it must apply in the case of a patient who is suicidal and has been hospitalised because of an overdose? Does respect for life here certainly imply respect for autonomy? I think we can say that there is scope for disagreement here and, more to the point, scope for the exercise of individual judgement.

Another area of potential disagreement in relation to the rule 'the patient's wishes must in all circumstances be respected' is where a patient's wish is for CPR when the physician judges CPR to be futile. The issue here might be put, crudely but clearly, in this way: is the physician simply providing a service, as a shopkeeper might, giving customers what they demand, or does professional integrity involve the exercise of judgement that may, in particular cases, legitimately resist a patient's request?

On this point, in relation to CPR, opinions differ. The guidelines adopted at Frenchay Hospital, Bristol, lay down that 'If at any time patients or their relatives request an attempt at resuscitation contrary to medical opinion – this should be carried out' (Baskett 1991). On the other hand, the Honorary Secretary of the Resuscitation Council (U.K.) has written as follows: 'The decision to initiate CPR should only be taken after asking ourselves the following questions: Does the patient want to be resuscitated? If the attempt is successful, will prolongation of life be in the patient's best interests? Can the underlying cause of the cardiac or respiratory arrest be reversed? If the answer to any one of these questions is no then we should not interfere with the process of dying'. (Handley 1990).

Here, what the patient wants is not held to be a sufficient condition for resuscitation and should not, in the author's opinion, over-ride medical judgement. An implication of this view appears to be that, in cases where the physician holds that CPR would be futile, consultation with patients and relatives in order to ascertain and take account of their views, is not appropriate, at best they should be informed of his or her decision. This is the view taken by Tomlinson and Brody (1988) 'When the absence of medical benefit is the rationale for a DNR order, communication with the patient or family should aim at securing an understanding of the decision the physician has already made. Eliciting the patient's values or involving the family in the decision is not required because the decision is based on medical expertise'.

Perhaps what is particularly at issue here is the question, what constitutes professional integrity? If a medical judgement is overridden by a moral judgement (for example, that patients' wishes ought to be respected), is this a loss or an expression of integrity?

The above discussion illustrates the need for a potentially complex process of decision-making in individual cases, in which all morally relevant factors are taken into account. This in turn suggests that, while there may be a need for guidelines to shape decision-making, strict generally applicable *rules* which short-circuit this process are inappropriate.

The view that guidelines are morally preferable to rules that must apply regardless, and that there must be space for the exercise of individual judgement, can be applied to such widespread rules as 'Always resuscitate in the absence of a DNR order', 'Always resuscitate within 24 hours of admission', and 'Always resuscitate within 24 hours after an operation'.

That judgement may be required in such cases is illustrated by the following comments from two experienced nurses:

Having worked with the very elderly undergoing major surgery for trauma fractures, the following has been known to occur. Because the patient is not more than 24 hours post-op, crash procedure is started. It is started even though everyone knows the patient is unlikely to survive, and the anaesthetist will call a halt almost as soon as he arrives and sees the age of the patient. Knowing all of this, it seems very unfair on the patient to subject them to resuscitation, knowing it would be to no avail.

I have found it distressing and morally worrying when I have had to resuscitate 'over 90s' post surgery, when they have had so many serious complications that it is clearly of no use. It seemed to me such an undignified and cruel end. These situations have occurred immediately post-op when policy dictated we must attempt resuscitation . . .

If the 24-hour rules are understood as guidelines and not as hard and fast rules, space is left to acknowledge the professional and moral propriety of individual judge ment.

Individual judgement

The notion of individual judgement is ambiguous. It may denote exercise of judgement by an individual, or the exercise of judgement in individual cases. This distinction has practical importance for decisions about resuscitation.

As regards the exercise of judgement by individual nurses, we have seen that even though it may be morally justified (as Ellis [1987] illustrates) it may be professionally risky. However, when an exercise of individual judge-ment is an attempt to 'act always in such a manner as to promote and safeguard the interests and wellbeing of patients and clients', a requirement central to the nurses' *Code of Professional Conduct* (UKCC 1992), there would be a prima facie obligation on the nurses' professional body to support their conscientious action.

What is at issue is the notion of professional integrity: if the role of the nurse were conceived of as simply instrumental, as simply that of carrying out orders, 'breaking the rules' would, in terms of role-morality at least, be hard to defend. But it is, of course, not conceived of in this way, as the *Code of Professional Conduct* (UKCC 1992) and recent emphasis on the nurse as patient advocate illustrate.

It is, of course, the case that the settled structure of care in hospitals necessarily involves nurses in implementing decisions made by medical staff, and since a settled structure is necessary for good patient care, it is desirable that individual decisions in relation to resuscitation by nurses should be exceptional.

One way of avoiding the necessity for such decisions is through prior collaborative discussion. The case for this must now be considered.

Collaboration

The UKCC *Code of Professional Conduct* (1992) lays down the duty that nurses should 'work in a collaborative . . . manner with other health care professionals'. But how far is collaboration possible in relation to decisions about resuscitation? And how far is it appropriate?

As to how far it is possible, this clearly depends on such contingent factors as the attitude, beliefs and personality of the consultant, since he or she has the power to determine how decisions are taken.

That it is appropriate follows from the earlier claim that decisions about resuscitation are essentially moral, not technically expert, decisions. Since, as has been shown, we are in the area of moral decision-making, discussion allows scope for differing moral perceptions to be voiced and tested. Since moral perceptions do not gain or lose validity by virtue of the status of those who put them forward, there is scope for the views of all members of the team, from the most junior nurse to the consultant, to be heard. Such discussion also allows for the expression of particular worries over aspects of policy in relation to individual patients, and hence can reduce the isolation of members of the team. It potentially minimises worry and dissatisfaction. (One nurse described her experience of no collaboration as follows: 'The doctors tend to make decisions, leaving nurses and other health care workers feeling unsatisfied and worried about decisions'.) It may also reduce the likelihood of situations arising in which nurses feel obliged to take lonely, professionally risky, decisions to go against whatever rules are in force, since policy in relation to individual patients will have been talked through within the team. Finally, of course, it provides a forum in which nurses are able to act as advocates for their patients.

This view, which associates affirmation of the right and duty of doctors to decide with the need for consultation and collaboration, is clearly expressed in the following extracts from an essay by Dunstan (Dunstan and Shinebourne 1989). In advocating the 'location of clinical decision in one identifiable individual, the doctor who accepts responsibility for the patient', Professor Dunstan acknowledges that 'decision is the culmination of a corporate process in which information and assessment are shared', and claims that 'decision is taken but consideration is shared. As each participant — nurse, laboratory scientist, junior doctor, social worker — is responsible for information or assessment professionally offered, so the consultant . . . accepts responsibility for the conclusion, the resultant decision, and is accountable for it'.

How Should Decisions be Communicated?

In a discussion of ethical issues relating to CPR, you may feel that reference to how decisions are communicated is out of place, for unlike the questions 'What would be justifiable grounds for giving or withholding CPR?' and 'Who should have the right to decide?', this may seem to be a purely procedural matter, a matter perhaps of health care standards of practice, but not of ethics.

The relation between standards of practice and ethics is interestingly discussed by Chadwick (1991). Here it is perhaps sufficient to note that how decisions are communicated can have a bearing on the interests and welfare of patients and also on the interests and welfare of staff. Bad communication can lead to misunderstanding, stress and patient abuse through CPR being mistakenly administered. Procedures, therefore, at least in this context, have moral implications and are appropriately a matter for moral evaluation.

That stress, confusion, and CPR being administered against the wishes of a patient can occur through decisions being communicated verbally is illustrated in the following comment, in which a nurse recalls her experience:

> Problems can arise if the doctor expressing a verbal wish is not on call, for example if the patient in question arrests. It is distressing to find yourself in the position of aiding in a 'resus' attempt that you know is against a decision taken by another doctor, and occasionally patients or relatives, just because the wrong person is available at the wrong time.

Another nurse highlights the insecurity attaching to verbal messages:

> Some other patients, deemed to be incurable, may have verbal messages about their inappropriateness for CPR

passed on by the medical staff. But as even the most junior nurse knows, one cannot afford to accept third- or fourth-hand oral communications, especially when they apply to something as serious as life itself.

One reason why nurses 'cannot afford' to accept such communications about withholding CPR is that, legally, a failure to resuscitate, causing death, is an omission that might give rise to charges of negligence, or even man-slaughter if it is claimed there has been gross negligence. Where there is the uncertainty that attaches to verbal messages, the pressure of this threat may well be a factor leading to CPR being initiated against a doctor's decision, and to the patient's detriment.

Concern about possible legal come-back is no doubt a motive behind verbal 'slow-code' orders. A nurse com-ments that in her experience 'there is often a verbal dis-crepancy to written notes — eg 'take a slow walk'. In other words, should the patient arrest, CPR is not officially withheld, and nurses are expected only to go through the motions. It is hard not to see this as an erosion of a nurse's professional dignity; it certainly implicates the nurse in an essentially dishonest practice — the nurse is being asked to participate in a sham treatment. It is also hard, therefore, not to see it as a practice which nurses would be justified in resisting and, indeed, in seeking to have abolished.

Whatever the content, verbal communications are clearly unsatisfactory. On this, Canham and Gunga (1985) can have the last, summarising, word: 'we should know from experience that verbal messages have no place in our vast, multi-disciplinary hospitals'.

Decisions, then, must be documented. How they are documented also has ethical implications. Canham and Gunga claim that 'written statements, in acceptable code if necessary, should be placed in every case note and every care plan'. This invites the question, why should code be 'necessary' and what would be 'acceptable'?

The use of code (for example, 'no 222', DNR, NFR or a star) may be in order that decisions not to resuscitate should remain covert, hidden both from patients and their relatives, in order to preclude any possible legal complications. If this is the motivation, it clearly runs counter to such principles as honesty and respect for autonomy. With the development of primary nursing, it also runs counter to moves by nurses to encourage patients to read and contribute to their care plans, and to ask for clarification of terms they do not understand.

Code may of course be regarded as 'necessary' simply as a matter of convenience. What might be 'acceptable' code? In the experience of some (Donnelly 1987), the practice of communicating 'Do not resuscitate' decisions by the code 'DNR' may have unfortunate consequences, in particular the consequence that patients so designated may be denied access to other measures, such as intensive care, artificial feeding and elective surgery. In one view, 'DNR' may come to be used as an adjective ('A DNR patient'), thus placing very different patients in the same category, with damaging implications for their treatment.

For these reasons, one hospital (Donnelly 1987) has abandoned the designation 'DNR' and adopted in its place the phrase 'no emergency CPR'. It is argued that this 'makes clearer the distinction between (1) emergency cardiopulmonary resuscitation and (2) intensive care and advanced life support provided on a selective basis'. It is also harder to abbreviate, and impossible to use as an adjective, thus removing the worry about labelling.

The worry that 'DNR' may be, on its own, too blunt an instrument has led one hospital (Townsend et al 1990) to identify four DNR categories. These are:

(1) DNR/maintain emergency drug protocols;

(2) DNR/no emergency drug protocols;
(3) DNR/comfort care only;
(4) DNR/other.

Category 3 is for those who are clearly dying and for whom aggressive therapy would be useless. Category 4 may be used by a physician to communicate about a special situation not covered by the other three orders.

What categories are appropriate or necessary is clearly a matter of expertise (although, as has been suggested, not a matter that is immune from moral comment). The general, ethical, point in relation to the communication of decisions to members of the health care team is surely this: whatever clarity is necessary to avoid patient abuse (through the use or withholding of CPR which goes against either the patient's condition or wishes, or both), and to minimise the emotional and moral costs to the health care team, should be sought.

Conclusion

CPR has developed as a powerful emergency technique that can restore patients to full, personal life, bringing them back from a death that is otherwise certain. It also has its dark side, as has been amply illustrated in this discussion. Unsurprisingly, therefore, as was indicated at the outset, it is an area of professional practice that is a source of much ethical concern.

The aim here has been to explore some of what seem to be the main issues that it raises, rather than to prescribe conclusions. However, certain conclusions have emerged in the course of the discussion which may perhaps usefully be summarised.

• Decisions about resuscitation should relate to individual patients, and not to categories of patient (eg the over 60s).

- Relevant criteria are the patient's wishes, the patient's condition and the patient's quality of life. The patient's age is not a morally relevant criterion, except insofar as it may bear on his or her condition and capacity to tolerate CPR.
- In principle, patients' wishes should be sought, although in particular cases it may not be possible to find out what they are. Since this is an area of great sensitivity, the paramount importance of the relationship between nurse and patient is indicated.
- As in other aspects of patient care, this involves adequate staffing levels, and raises questions of resources. It is thus a particular area in which advocacy on behalf of patients is indicated.
- Although decision-taking is ultimately a medical responsibility, collaboration between all members of the health care team is of paramount importance. Where this is not the case, members of the health care team have an obligation to attempt to establish such collaboration.
- Although patient care in relation to resuscitation requires rules, these should be envisaged as guidelines, in order to validate the moral and professional propriety of individual judgment which may, from time to time, require that the 'rules' be broken.
- All decisions regarding resuscitation should be documented.
- 'Slow-code' instructions, whether verbal or documented in code, should be regarded as unethical.

I am especially indebted to Meta Muncaster and Breda Gibson for help and encouragement in reflecting on this topic, and to Breda Gibson, Catherine Cain, Chrissie Dunn and Caroline Shuldham for commenting on a first draft. Also to students in the Community Studies department of Reading University, for sharing their nursing experience of CPR with me.

References

Baskett, P.J.F. (1991) The ethics of resuscitation. In Evans, T.R. (ed) The ABC of Resuscitation (2nd ed). *British Medical Journal*, London.

Bayer, A.J., Ang, B.C. and Pathy, M.S.J. (1985) Cardiac arrests in a geriatric unit. *Age and Ageing*, **14**: 271–6.

Bedell, S.E. and Delbanco, T.L. (1984) Choices about cardiopulmonary resuscitation in hospital: when do physicians talk with patients? *New England Journal of Medicine*, **310** (17): 1089–93.

Blackhall, L.J. (1987) Must we always use CPR? *New England Journal of Medicine*, **317** (20): 1281–5.

Bleich, J.D. (1989) The moral obligation of the physician in the rabbinic tradition. In Dunstan G.R. and Shinebourne E.A. (eds.), *Doctors' Decisions*, Oxford, Oxford University Press.

Candy, C.E. (1991) 'Not for resuscitation': the student nurses' viewpoint, *Journal of Advanced Nursing*, **16**: 138–46.

Canham, J. and Gunga D. (1985) A matter of life or death. *Nursing Times*, **81**, (46): 52.

Chadwick, R.F. (1991) Is there a difference between standards and ethics? *Journal of Advances in Health and Nursing Care*, **1** (1): 75–89.

Dolan, M.B. (1988) Coding abuses hurt nurses, too. *Nursing*, **18** (2):47.

Donnelly, W.J. (1987) DNR: the case for early retirement. *Archives of Internal Medicine*, **147** (1): 38.

Dunstan, G.R. and Shinebourne, E.A., (eds.) (1989) *Doctor's Decisions, Ethical Conflicts in Medical Practice*. Oxford, Oxford University Press.

Ellis, K. (1987) The slow code dilemma. *Registered Nurse*, **50**, June: 28–9.

Evans, A.L. and Brody, B.A. (1985) The do-not-resuscitate

order in teaching hospitals. *Journal of American Medical Association*, **253**, (15): 2236–9.

Farber, N.J., Weiner, J.L. and Boyer, E.J. (1985) Cardiopulmonary resuscitation. Values and decisions — a comparison of health care professions. *Medical Care*, **23** (12): 1391–8.

Fusgen, I. and Summar, J.D. (1978) How much sense is there in an attempt to resuscitate an aged person? *Gerontology*, **24** (1): 37–45.

Gaskell, M. (1977) An investigation into the problems of deciding which hospital patients are/are not to be resuscitated. Unpublished MSc dissertation. University of Manchester.

Gunasekera, N.P.R., Tiller, D.J. and Clements, L.T-J. (1986) Elderly patients' views on cardiopulmonary resuscitation. *Age and Ageing*, **15**: 364–8.

Handley, A.J. (1990) Should we resuscitate? *Care of the Critically Ill*, **6** (4): 152–3.

Health Service Commissioner (1991) *Annual Report for 1990–1991*. London, HMSO.

Johnson, A.L., Tanser, P.H. and Ulan, R.A. (1967) Results of cardiac resuscitation in 552 patients. *American Journal of Cardiology*, **20**: 831–5.

Kass, L.R. (1980) Ethical dilemmas in the care of the ill: What is the good of the patient? *Journal of the American Medical Association*, **244** (17): 1949–9.

Kübler-Ross, E. (1969) *On Death and Dying*. New York, Macmillan.

Murphy, D.J., Murray, A.M. and Robinson, B.E. (1989) Outcomes of cardiopulmonary resuscitation in the elderly. *Annals of Internal Medicine*, **111**: 199–205.

Nolan, K. (1987) In death's shadow: the meanings of withholding resuscitation. *Hastings Center Report*, Oct/Nov: 9–14.

Nursing Times (1966) Resuscitation — the nurse's responsibility. **62**, Nov 11: 1497.

Nursing Times (1983) SRN said she chose to let man 'die peacefully'. **79** (19): 19.

O'Neill, O. (1984) Paternalism and partial autonomy. *Journal of Medical Ethics*, **10** (4): 173–8.

Peatfield, R.C., Taylor, D. and Sillet, R.W. (1977) Survival after cardiac arrest in hospital. *The Lancet*, **1**: 1223–5.

Schade, S.G. and Muslin, H. (1989) Do not resuscitate decisions: discussions with patients. *Journal of Medical Ethics*, **15** (4): 186–190.

Stewart, K. and Rai, G. (1985) A matter of life and death *Nursing Times*, **85** (35): 27–9.

Tomlinson, T. and Brody, H. (1988) Ethics and communication in do-not-resuscitate orders. *New England Journal of Medicine*, **318** (1): 43–46.

Townsend, M.B., Vass, B.C. and Defontes, J. (1990) Clarifying resuscitation status: a new approach. *Nursing Management*, **21** (10): 88a.

UKCC (1992) *Code of Professional Conduct* (3rd edn.) London, UKCC.

Wachter, R.M., Luce, J.M., Herst, N. and Lo, B. (1989) Decisions about resuscitation: inequities among patients with different diseases but similar prognoses. *Annals of Internal Medicine*, **111**: 525–32.

CHAPTER 4

Euthanasia

Verena Tschudin

Euthanasia should be a 'good death'. Judging by the debate surrounding the subject, it may be more a question of avoiding a bad death — a situation which perhaps medicine has created for itself.

Euthanasia — like all other ethical issues — concerns people who are in relationships. One person's right is another's responsibility. But is one person's right to die another person's responsibility to kill? Contradictions at all levels of this debate are addressed in this chapter, leading not necessarily to conclusions, but probably to further questions and further discussions.

The personal and social values most questioned are those which infringe on life — the making, taking and keeping of it. Because the issues are far from clear-cut, they cause personal and social problems. They fascinate and disgust; people are attracted to them and repelled by them; they judge them and are being judged by them.

Euthanasia — like all the other topics in this volume — is too large a subject to be covered entirely in one chapter. Some aspects can, however, be addressed, at least in the way of presenting them for further thought and discussion.

The Value of Life

Most ethical systems have some injunction against killing. 'Thou shalt not kill' is perhaps the best-known Western injunction. Some modern translations of the Bible, however, render this as 'Do not commit murder', thereby giving this instruction a different emphasis, and one which is more easily applicable in the setting of this chapter.

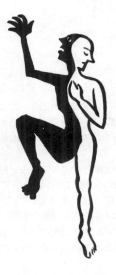

Another formulation has been made by Thiroux (1977) when he says that 'Human beings should revere life and accept death' (p. 124).

Life is that which is essentially given. 'There is an element of sheer mystery about human existence which lays a claim upon men (sic) to reverence and respect it, to foster it and not to destroy it' (Mahoney 1984, p. 41). What all people have in common is life, and therefore the reverence of life is a universal value, but not an absolute one. People and nations have always regarded their lives as (more) valuable and those of aliens and racial minorities as comparatively less valuable. In the past societies have tolerated duels and sacrificial killings, while wars, capital punishment, suicide, killing in self-defence and abortion are present infringements on life and its value.

If it is not possible to value or respect all life equally and universally, it must be asked whose life — or which life — is to be valued? Who decides? And on what basis?

The traditional doctrine of the *sanctity of life* is applied to *human* life only, and its proponents claim that all human life is of equal worth. Therefore the life of someone suffering from intractable pain and physical and mental agony, the life of a mass murderer and the life of a baby born with multiple deformities are all equally worthy, equally sacred, and should all be preserved. Life is not valuable because of its qualities, but is valuable in itself.

It could be argued that this is somewhat hypocritical, and today people are becoming much more aware of the value of *all* life, plants, animals and the universe as a whole included. It is not acceptable any more to say that only human life is sacred; indeed, some animals seem to live worthier lives than humans, and ants, for instance, form at least as well organised a society as humans do. Should the lives of ants and humans be of equal worth? This is not as absurd as it may sound, and the members of the Jain faith, a non-Brahminical Hindu sect, certainly hold to this ideal.

In order to appreciate the value of life it has been argued that some people are *innocent*, and their lives are worthy of preservation. Among these would normally be the sick and dying of any age. Those who are not innocent, such as criminals and perverts of any kind, cannot expect to have their lives valued as highly. This argument concludes that *killing* innocent people is wrong and therefore prohibited, but killing the non-innocent is not.

A further distinction needs to be made between *intentional* and *non-intentional* killing. Clearly it is wrong to kill a person intentionally, but not so wrong to kill non-intentionally. But where does the dividing line lie? This is a very important point when considering euthanasia and many of the debates on the subject hang on it. Giving someone a lethal injection is certainly intentional killing, but giving someone narcotics for pain is laudable even though that person may die from either increasing addiction or inability to maintain function.

Without necessarily using these words or ideas, nurses have long concerned themselves with the distinction between quality and quantity of life, particularly with respect to dying patients. This is a simple measure which is valid enough until it comes to a decision: who decides when quantity has reached its limit, or what is 'quality' under the circumstances?

It is often easy to hold an opinion simply because it seems 'right' without ever having followed the argument through. People tend to trust either their intuition or a particular argument, yet still never follow either to the end. In the area of the distinctions between innocence and non-innocence, between intentionally and non-intentionally killing someone, there are many debates raging. In his book *The End of Life* Rachels (1986) sets out to debunk these distinctions. He argues that every one of these theories, when taken to its logical conclusion, fails to be convincing. He shows that it is possible that any traditional ways of looking at life, killing, innocence and their opposites need only a little debate and they cannot stand up.

The most obvious example of the distinction between killing and murder is perhaps found in the area of euthanasia. This has been shown by the many cases where relatives 'helped' a person to die and when brought to law were either acquitted or sentenced lightly. The juries in these cases did not see this as murder, and the circumstances of the dying person and the relative seemed to suggest that in cases other than 'innocence' as traditionally seen, killing is also accepted as possible.

To show that these theories can be debunked, Rachels starts from a completely different standpoint. He believes that there:

is a deep difference between *having a life* and merely *being alive.* . . . Being alive, in the biological sense, is relatively unimportant. One's (biographical) life, by contrast, is immensely important; it is the sum of one's aspirations, decisions, activities, projects and human relationships. (p. 5)

If this is taken as a starting-point, the concepts and practicalities of euthanasia also start differently and certainly end differently. Rachels' ideas have been and are widely debated, both for and against; this work is referred to throughout this chapter.

Euthanasia in History

As euthanasia is a concept and a word with a specific history, it will be helpful to trace its path briefly.

The Greeks, whose language gave the word euthanasia (*eu* = good; *thanatos* = death) to the world, took a different attitude towards human life than we have today. Infanticide was openly required for deformed or unhealthy babies in Sparta, and while in Athens it was not a requirement, it was nevertheless the practice. The Greeks were also well known for their system of city-states which condemned anyone from outside such a state to a life of drudgery and often slavery.

Various examples can be quoted from throughout the world of the treatment of the elderly and infirm:

When an elderly Aymara Indian from Bolivia becomes terminally ill his relatives and friends keep a vigil beside him. If death comes slowly, he may ask for assistance in dying, and then the family will withhold food and drink until he slips into unconsciousness. In some Eskimo cultures too, when an old person is ready for death he will ask his family to help him on his way. (Kennedy 1990, p. 15)

The idea of euthanasia has become notorious in its use by the Nazis in some of their practices. The seeds of this were sown in the early part of the century, and in 1920 a book with the title *Permitting the Destruction of Lives Not Worth Living* was published. It later became evident that about half of all German mental hospital patients had died of starvation or infectious illnesses during World War I. The connection to racial hygiene was easy, and this gradually led to ways of eliminating Jews, gypsies, homosexuals, the mentally ill and anyone labelled not worthy of living.

The word 'euthanasia' had become a euphemism for murderous practices of many kinds, but by using that word it could be seen as something humanitarian and benign. It was only at the Nuremberg Trials in 1947 that many of the machinations and experiments — mostly carried out by doctors — came to light. 'The meaning of Nazi "euthanasia" can be understood only in the context of their especially virulent kind of racism' (Rachels 1986, p. 177). Hitler had accepted that there is such a thing as a life not worth living — as many humanitarians also have — but for Hitler this meant a life that could not form part of the 'Volk' — the German people.

Rachels makes the point strongly that 'contemporary proponents of euthanasia advocate mercy-killing in response to the patient's request'. For the Nazis, however, there were never 'any thoughts of securing the permission of the victims. The sterilisations as well as the killings were completely involuntary' (p. 178).

This distinction, nevertheless, does not seem to cut much ice in the German-speaking world today. In 1989 there were protests in several places in Germany where lectures were to be given by Peter Singer, Director of the Centre for Human Bioethics, Monash University, Melbourne, on 'Bio-engineering, ethics and mental disability'. Protests were also reported in Austria in 1990 and

1991, and Switzerland in 1991 (*Bulletin of Medical Ethics* nos. 61, 63, 69 and 70) when similar lectures were to be given. The collective memory and instinctive fear seem stronger than rational arguments.

Definitions

Following on from the above, it is clear that definitions of euthanasia are very important.

In the Linacre Centre Working Party Report *Euthanasia and Clinical Practice* (1982), the following definition is used:

> There is *euthanasia* when the death of a human being is brought about on purpose as part of the medical care being given him. (p. 2)
>
> That range of use of the term 'euthanasia' for which the notion of benefit is critical, stakes out the central subject matter of [the] enquiry.

Accordingly, the brief definition above can be expanded as follows:

> in euthanasia a person's death is brought about on the ground that, because of his present or likely future mental condition and quality of life (and sometimes in consideration too of the quality of life of his family) it would be better for him (or at least no harm) if that person were dead. (p. 3)

Beauchamp and Davidson (1979) argue that five conditions must be satisfied for an act to be called euthanasia:

- Death must be intended.
- There must be conscious pain, mental anguish and/ or serious self-burdensomeness.
- Death-causing acts must be motivated by beneficence, and the means of death must not cause more suffering.

- Any death act must be as painless and merciful as possible.
- There must be non-fetal humanity (to distinguish between abortion and euthanasia).

There are four recognised types of euthanasia:

- Voluntary — the patient freely chooses death and may ask for help with dying.
- Involuntary — death is caused without the person's consent and may even be imposed against that person's wishes or desires.
- Active — this involves the deliberate act which causes death.
- Passive — this involves a deliberate omission or withholding of certain life-supporting treatments.

Thus four categories of euthanasia are recognised:

- Voluntary active euthanasia
- Voluntary passive euthanasia
- Involuntary active euthanasia
- Involuntary passive euthanasia

Voluntary active euthanasia generally means that a person who is critically ill asks to have her or his life actively ended, ie with an overdose or death-inducing drug, or by switching off life-support equipment.

Voluntary passive euthanasia means on the whole that a person asks that no more treatments be given and that he or she be allowed to die of the consequences of disease or illness.

Involuntary active euthanasia applies when a person, whom others regard as needlessly suffering, is given a death-inducing drug or has life-support equipment switched off.

Involuntary passive euthanasia means that a person who seems to be suffering or leading an otherwise 'senseless' life in a coma or other vegetative state is not treated any further in crucial situations.

The distinction is therefore made between euthanasia (active voluntary and active involuntary) and *letting people die* (passive voluntary and passive involuntary euthanasia). Letting people die is then seen simply as good medical practice. Others, however, have argued that letting someone die when the life could be saved is still euthanasia. Rachels (1986) highlights the difference rather starkly when he says:

> There is nothing wrong with being the cause of
> someone's death if his death is, all things considered, a
> good thing. And if his death is *not* a good thing, then
> no form of euthanasia, active or passive, is justified.
> (p. 115)

He goes on to say that 'our duty not to harm people is generally more stringent than our duty to help them'. Thus letting someone critically ill die is generally all right, while standing by and letting someone who could be saved die is not, although it can still technically be called letting die.

This leads to a further distinction being applied: that between 'ordinary' and 'extraordinary' means.

The sanctity of life principle — mainly a Roman Catholic view — accepts that life is God-given, and that a patient should do everything to maintain his or her life. Therefore in certain circumstances a patient is *obliged* to accept treatments. The *value of life* principle, however, takes a wider humanitarian view, and here both patient and doctor need to consider when treatment is obligatory or indicated, and if so, which kind of treatment.

Ordinary means (of treatment) refer to normal and tried procedures, whereas *extraordinary* means refer to:

> an unusual procedure, involving much risk, pain or heavy cost. The fact that a treatment is in this sense 'ordinary' is itself a reason for holding it to be normally obligatory, though there may be circumstances in which this reason lacks force; for example, when one considers the use of antibiotics for pneumonia in a patient in the terminal phase of another illness. (Linacre Centre 1982, p. 45)

This last point shows how difficult it is to maintain any rules of ethics or morality because they can always be seen to fail at some stage. Morality always happens at the fringe, between the acceptable and the not (yet) acceptable. Thus while today a heart transplant may still come into the category of 'extraordinary' means for saving life, this may change in a few years and be an ordinary means, like antibiotics once were.

Another definition to be made in this debate is that of *intention*. In this setting it means that for the term euthanasia to apply, death has to be *intended*. Campbell and Collinson (1988) say that 'when we know the intention with which someone acts we know both the point of the action and something about the person who acts'. Thus it can be seen that the intentional killing of innocent humans has come to be the basis for the Churches to condemn abortion, suicide and euthanasia. But, argues Rachels (1986), if the sanctity of life principle is strictly applied, soldiers and criminals should also come under that principle. Is the intention *killing* or helping?

Euthanasia or Suicide?

Ever since Socrates, who was condemned to death by drinking a cup of hemlock at sunset, insisted that he drink it before the appointed hour, the question has been whether this was execution or suicide. And did Captain Oates, a member of the group who accompanied Scott on his last expedition to the South Pole, commit suicide by going out in the blizzard? Did he kill himself, or did the blizzard kill him?

The point has been made that a condemned man's walk to the scaffold might, therefore, also be called suicide. But Campbell and Collinson (1988) point out that this is not correct. Only if the condemned man would also press the switch that operates the device that kills him, could he also be described as his own executioner (p. 11).

Thiroux (1977) compared active voluntary euthanasia (he calls it 'mercy death') with *assisted suicide*. He says that 'terminally ill patients are often unable to commit suicide and therefore ask someone to "put them out of their misery". These patients not only give their permission to end their lives, but also, in most cases, request or even demand that their lives be terminated' (p. 172).

Camus (1955) said that 'there is but one truly philosophical problem and that is suicide'. Suicide has been decriminalised in Britain since 1961 but 'it is still an offence to aid and abet suicide and survivors of suicide pacts may be prosecuted' (Duncan et al 1977, p. 425). The suicide which is linked to euthanasia is of a particular kind in that it always happens in conditions of extreme physical suffering. It is argued, therefore, that what such a person has the right to do on his own (ie bring about his own death), he also has the right to ask someone to help him do as long as there is no coercion and no third party's rights are violated. Rachels (1986) argues that if suicide is permissible, it is clear that with these provisos, euthanasia is also permissible.

Cases of assisted suicide happen in hospitals and at

home. Saving up certain tablets and then taking them all at once is perhaps still the most common form of this type of death. This may involve a close friend or relative who will then help the patient to swallow the tablets all at once. This type of death is, however, usually furtive, and *may* be painful and uncomfortable.

A curious case of assisted suicide was reported in 1990. Dr Jack Kevorkian (*Bulletin of Medical Ethics*, 62, p. 20), a retired pathologist in Michigan, invented a 'suicide machine'. This consisted of a saline drip which, when a red button was pressed, changed the infusion to a sedative, followed a minute later by potassium chloride. Kevorkian had used his machine on a 54-year-old woman from Oregon who had sought his help, having been diagnosed as being in the early stages of Alzheimer's disease. Once she had pressed the red button she died within five minutes. Murder charges were initially brought against Kevorkian but then dropped (*Bulletin of Medical Ethics*, 65, p. 6) 'because the state of Michigan has no clear law against assisting suicide, so alternative charges could not be brought'.

In both suicide and euthanasia the intention is the death of the person. But according to Campbell and Collinson (1988) there is a difference between unequivocal suicide and a self-inflicted death of self-renunciation: between those who take their lives and those who give them (p. 6). There is a case for distinguishing 'between what a person intends in his action (the suicide) and the foreseen but unintended results of the action (the grief and probably guilt of those left behind), and it takes a person to intend both the end and the means of his action' (p. 7); for example, Captain Oates must have intended his death to free his companions from the burden of his presence. It is possible to see assisted suicide as such a 'giving' of life.

The Right to Die

Voluntary euthanasia rests heavily on the arguments that people have a right to choose, and in particular the right to choose death. This has become known as 'the right to die'. As well as arguing from autonomy, the right to die rests on the notion of the rights to maintain dignity, to reduce suffering and to be treated fairly (Johnstone 1989, p. 254).

According to Miller (1987), to establish a 'right to die' is 'problematic because of the associations that *right* suggests with duties and obligations'. Miller compares the right to die with the right, acknowledged in America, to eat:

> If a person can no longer feed himself, then society has various duties and obligations to help him. In the same way, when it is time for that person to die, doctors have various duties and obligations to help him do so with his autonomy, and to replace technology by real people in dying situations — in the belief that when I am breathing my last breath, it is better to be touched by a hand than violated by a tube. I want the process of death taken out of the control of machines and returned to people.

The right to die is a more hotly debated issue in the USA where litigous medicine is common. Several famous cases have continued to be international news for years. Yet it was only in the Nancy Beth Cruzan case that the debate actually reached the Supreme Court (*Bulletin of Medical Ethics*, 60, p. 23). Cruzan, in her late twenties, had a car accident which left her in an unconscious state. After it became evident that she would not regain her mental faculties, her parents asked that the artificial nutrition and hydration be terminated. The employees at the hospital refused to do this as they knew it would cause her death. Various courts were involved, ruling, among other things, that her parents were not entitled to order the termination of her medical treatment. The whole issue is made more complicated in the USA by the fact that patients (or their relatives) have to pay for such treatments.

A similar case has been reported in the British press of a 20-year-old man who had been injured at the Hillsborough football stadium disaster in 1989. Two and a half years later his parents would like his intravenous feeding to be discontinued, but no-one is prepared to do this, and if the parents did it themselves they could be charged with attempted murder (*Daily Telegraph*, 31 August 1991).

The US President's Commission Report *Deciding to Forego Life-Sustaining Treatment* (1983) emphasised the importance of the following issues regarding dying patients' wishes (*Bulletin of Medical Ethics*, 38):

1 respecting the choices of individuals competent to decide to forego even life-sustaining treatment;
2 providing mechanisms and guidelines for decision-making on behalf of patients unable to do so on their own;
3 affirming a presumption in favour of sustaining life;
4 improving the medical options available to dying patients;
5 providing respectful, responsible, and supportive care to patients for whom no further medical therapies are available or elected; and
6 encouraging health care institutions to take responsibility for ensuring that adequate procedures for decision-making are available to patients.

These guidelines cover most of the ethical principles generally acknowledged, ie the value of life (3), beneficence (4), respect for the person (1), justice (5), truth-telling (2) and autonomy or individual freedom for patients and staff

(6). In this way the integrity of all concerned is not only maintained but also fostered.

The right to die mostly concerns patients who are conscious and 'competent', who can speak for themselves and argue for themselves. The matter is, however, completely different when it concerns someone unable to speak or decide. This will be considered after a short excursion into living wills.

Living Wills

'It seems unfair that I can make provision for what I want to happen *after* my death, but I cannot make provision for things that will certainly happen to me if my brain deteriorates *before* death' (Andrews 1989). This is the increasing argument of many people, and the reason why living wills have gained in popularity in recent years.

A living will, advance directives, or advance declaration, is a document which a person signs in the presence of two witnesses, and hands to her or his general practitioner. In the UK the form is supplied by the Voluntary Euthanasia Society, and is for *guidance only*: it is *not* a legal document. The USA had published its *Patient Self-Determination Act* in 1990 and accepts advance directives 'such as a living will or durable power of attorney for health care recognized under state law' (*Bulletin of Medical Ethics*, 65, p. 3). It has been suggested that by 1990 about 10 per cent of all US adults had already signed living wills, mostly influenced by the Cruzan case, and that with the new Act this figure may rise sharply.

There is a great difference between withdrawing treatment from a critically ill patient, and not embarking on any treatment in the first place. The living will makes it clear that those who sign it do not want any treatment started. They do not want to become 'sedated, comatose,

LIVING WILLS
GUIDANCE FOR NURSES

INTRODUCTION

Concern has been expressed by nurses at the growing prevalence of so-called living wills. This guidance has been produced in order to assist nurses to consider the ethical issues involved.

WHAT IS A LIVING WILL?

A living will is a document which attempts to set out the kind of health care that would be authorised by a patient who is unable to choose, for example because the patient is unconscious, or delirious, or otherwise incapacitated. It is an attempt to allow patients the right to refuse treatment in advance, in case the patient is too ill to choose for themselves or becomes unable to express that choice as their condition deteriorates.

WHAT DOES A LIVING WILL LOOK LIKE ?

Living wills have been produced by various groups in a format which usually includes the name of the patient and the signature. It may have been witnessed and countersigned. The document may seek to place a limit on treatment, or to authorise risky procedures.

You may first encounter a living will when the patient asks you to witness it, when you find it in the possession of a confused or unconscious patient, or when the patient gives it to you on admission to hospital.

In some cases, patients may simply have a letter with them stating what they want.

WHAT IS THE STRENGTH OF A LIVING WILL ?

The best care for patients always takes the patient's wishes into account.

The strength of the living will is that it allows the patient to make a statement which will still be there for people to read after the patient becomes too ill to repeat it. It would appear that the law is confused in this area and the decision whether to treat at the end of life often seems arbitrary.

A living will may increase patient choice.

WHAT IS THE WEAKNESS OF A LIVING WILL ?

The living will is not a recognised legal document in this country. You cannot tell the state of mind of the patient when the living will was signed or whether it was done under duress. The living will may be out of date.

Health care staff, like everyone else, are subject to the law which prohibits taking steps or giving advice that would assist another person to commit suicide.

It is difficult to draft a living will that is clear and unambiguous, and interpretations could differ.

Living wills may be a response to poor provision for health care, and may be viewed as a disincentive to improve care. For example if enough people stated that they would rather die than go into a nursing home, nursing homes would cease to exist.

ETHICAL DILEMMAS

Vulnerable or dying people have a right to know that their nurses will provide the best possible care, and will maintain their dignity, especially when they are unable to do this for themselves. An abrupt refusal to accept a living will might damage the trust that the patient has in the nurse.

Ethical dilemmas about treatment at the end of life are often made worse by poor communication. A nurse may wonder what lies behind the motives of medical staff or relatives who support the idea of not treating a patient. The nurse may feel that there is a duty to treat the patient if at all possible.

On the other hand the nurse may feel that treatment in the last stages of life is merely unthinking interference. This can only be resolved by a full discussion with as many of the people involved as possible.

WHAT SHOULD THE NURSE DO ABOUT LIVING WILLS ?

Junior staff cannot work without safe guidelines within their own clinical area. Nurses must press for clear local guidelines about when to initiate treatment of any patient.

For any patient, whether or not they have made a living will, it should be made quite clear who has been involved in the decision to withhold treatment from a patient who cannot consent or refuse.

Nurses should avoid signing or drawing up living wills for a patient. A legalistic document is no substitute for the sense of trust and security provided by a good nurse-patient relationship, within the multi-disciplinary setting.

Nurses must be aware of the way in which their own moral background influences their response to difficult decisions. Nurses need to develop communications skills so that they are able to raise questions about treatment with patients sensitively and are able to discuss dilemmas about treatment with the rest of the team.

Nurses must take an active part in making sure that the wishes of patients are taken into account when decisions about treatment at the end of life are made.

FURTHER READING

Age Concern The Living Will; Consent to treatment at the end of life, London, Edward Arnold, 1988

Kennedy I, Treat me Right - Essays in medical law and ethics, London, Clarendon Press, 1988

Rowson R, An introduction to Ethics for Nurses-, London, Scutari Press, 1990

Reprinted March 1992 Order No. 000 102

ROYAL COLLEGE OF NURSING

Issues in nursing and health

betubed objects, manipulated and subconscious, if not subhuman' (Fletcher 1977).

The argument against living wills tends to be that those who sign them do not then in the critical moment or circumstance have the possibility to change their mind. If they should be in an accident where it is obvious that a short time of life-saving treatments would give them good quality of life, they would then not be able to be treated. It is impossible to foresee how someone would feel and act later and therefore one could give away too much too early.

One possible way of safeguarding this is by giving durable power of attorney for health care to one (or two) close people. Age Concern (1988) recommended that if legislation were to be introduced, the two instruments could be combined. This:

'allows the directions of the living will to be general, setting the context within which the agent named in the durable power of attorney will be guided as to how best to make detailed decisions, in relation to the specific circumstances which arise in the particular case'. (p. 82)

Those people who are concerned that doctors base their 'decisions to treat or not to treat, on judgements about someone's worth as a human being' (Lockwood 1985) at a time when they do not know that person and his or her own values of life, and would be reassured that by this proposed measure the rights and values of the patient are respected. The duties and obligations of the caring team may, however, be challenged by this. It must be emphasised, though, that at the time of writing (1991) all this is speculation and probability and not legally binding.

The presence of a living will in the patient's case notes may render many a nurse uneasy, wondering what the relationship with the patient is: does the patient not trust the nurse's care?; can the nurse really *be* a carer in such a case? The RCN has published a document on the subject (figure 4.2), setting guidelines for nurses in such situations.

The 'Incompetent' Patient

The real 'crunch' with euthanasia comes when it is or is not practised on people who cannot, for one reason or another, speak for themselves. According to the Linacre Centre (1982, p. 51) there are three classes of *incompetent* patients:

1 those who were once competent (mostly the unconscious)
2 those who though physically mature have always been incompetent (mostly mentally ill people)
3 infants and young children

The particular difficulty for these patients is that they may be discriminated against and judged to be leading inferior lives. People who argue against euthanasia on the principle of the 'slippery slope' generally see the danger that if it is practised openly, it is easy to 'eliminate' various categories of people, especially those who cannot speak for themselves or defend themselves.

There is a long tradition that in the case of incompetence, any decisions are taken by relatives or guardians, on the grounds that they have the patient's best interests at heart, but this cannot be taken for granted. Indeed, in the case of Nancy Cruzan, the courts ruled that her parents could not decide for her.

The Linacre Centre (1982) argues that 'the basic standard in the treatment of the incompetent should be no different from that which holds for the competent, ie they should be given whatever treatment is beneficial, having

TO MY FAMILY AND MY PHYSICIAN

This declaration is made by me ....
    (full name and address)

....

....

at a time when I am of sound mind and after careful consideration.

If I am unable to take part in decisions about my medical care owing to my physical or mental incapacity and if I develop one or more of the medical conditions listed in Item Three below and two independent physicians conclude that there is no prospect of my recovery, I declare that my wishes are as follows:

1. I request that my life shall not be sustained by artificial means such as life support systems, intravenous fluids or drugs, or by tube feeding.

2. I request that distressing symptoms caused either by the illness or by lack of food or fluid should be controlled by appropriate sedative treatment, even though such treatment may shorten my life.

3. The said medical conditions are:

   (1) Severe and lasting brain damage sustained as a result of injury, including stroke, or disease.

   (2) Advanced disseminated malignant disease.

   (3) Advanced degenerative disease of the nervous and/or muscular systems with severe limitations of independent mobility, and no satisfactory response to treatment.

   (4) Senile or pre-senile dementia e.g. Alzheimer or multi-infarct type.

   (5) Other condition of comparable gravity.

*Cross out and initial any condition you do not wish to include.

I further declare that I hereby absolve my medical attendants from any civil liability arising from action taken in response to and in terms of this Declaration.

I reserve my right to revoke this Declaration at any time.

Signature: ....

Date: ....

Witnessed by:

Signature: ....   Signature: ....

Name: ....   Name: ....
    (please print)   (please print)

Address: ....   Address: ....

....

....

....

regard to acceptable costs in terms of expense and burden' (p. 50). But the same Report cites the case of a patient in the US, a 67-year-old profoundly mentally retarded man who had been institutionalised all his life and was unable to communicate verbally. He developed acute myeloblastic leukaemia, which is normally treated with chemotherapy but has a poor prognosis. In view of the side effects of chemotherapy (discomfort, anaemia, bladder irritation, loss of hair and bone marrow depression) it was felt that this man could not tolerate this treatment, as he would probably be unable to cooperate with it.

The care of newborn infants with malformations or physical or mental handicaps is a perennial problem. The famous case of Dr Leonard Arthur made headlines in 1981, when he ordered that a newborn infant with Down's syndrome — whose parents had rejected him on that account at birth — be given 'nursing care only'. In effect this meant that he was given DF118 at the discretion of the nurse in charge but not more than every four hours, and water only (p. 85). The baby died a few days later. Dr Arthur was charged with murder, but acquitted.

The care of incompetent patients who are critically ill is the most problematic with regard to euthanasia. The questions asked at the beginning of this chapter (Who decides? And on what basis?) are the most pressing in these situations. There are no laws giving instructions, and the health carers' Codes of Conduct invariably exhort them to preserve life. In such situations it is, therefore, often their Code which wins because it is the health carer's values which are immediately questioned. The instinct to protect themselves is overriding the instinct to care for others.

With increasing technology it is possible to prolong life, but many people ask, what sort of life will it become?

Kennedy (1990) recounts the case of Mr Kahn, a patient of Dr Christiaan Barnard, the pioneer in heart-transplant surgery:

Aged 78, Mr Kahn had cancer of the prostate, obstruction of the bowel and severe emphysema. On admission to hospital he told the consultant quite calmly that he no longer wished to live, but the consultant told him that, in accordance with practice, his condition would be treated.

The man in the bed next to Mr Kahn was suffering from inoperable stomach cancer and was totally unconscious with tubes connected to his abdomen, lungs and bladder. One day he had a heart attack which brought the resuscitation unit hurrying to his bedside. 'They did not know why his heart had arrested,' said Dr Barnard, 'and what quality of life he could be given if his heart was restarted. Their sole purpose was to restart the heart. They jumped on the old man, they massaged his heart from the outside, they shocked him and they ventilated his lungs.' To no avail: the man died. And Mr Kahn said to the consultant, 'Doctor, please promise that you will never let that happen to me, because I am a proud man and I do not fear death.' The consultant said nothing.

A few days later Mr Kahn developed problems with his lungs and they put a tube down his windpipe and connected him to a mechanical respirator to keep him alive; there was nothing he could do about it because he was now too weak to resist.

'That night', continued Dr Barnard, 'when the nurse looked at Mr Kahn, she could see that the respirator was doing his breathing for him and that the monitor showed that his heart was beating. But in the morning Mr Kahn was dead. During the night he had managed to disconnect the respirator; and on the bed there was a note, written in a shaky hand. 'Doctor, the real enemy is not death — it is inhumanity'. (pp. 7–9)

This story, while not of an incompetent person, still shows that treatments can render a person 'incompetent'.

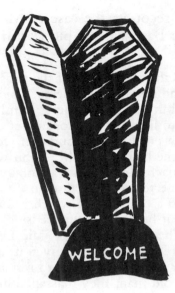

The point, however, is that 'the enemy is inhumanity'. And the question is, what is inhumanity — or humanity — in such situations? Is it to treat, or to let die? This will shortly be discussed — after one more aspect is considered.

'Nursing Care Only'

Rachels (1986) believes that doctors traditionally have three options when faced with a seriously ill patient: 'First, they can end his life now by a lethal injection. Second, they can withhold treatment and allow him to die sooner than he otherwise would. . . . And third, they could continue treatment and prolong his life as long as possible' (p. 108).

However, Rachels is a Professor of Philosophy and has

presumably never seen a prescription chart for a terminally ill person with the words 'Nursing care only'
written on it. Doctors can in truth withhold treatment —
their treatment — but this still leaves a patient in bed to
be cared for.

Johnstone (1989) is scathing in her attack on this directive. She believes that when doctors argue that euthanasia
is not needed because the *medical profession* has been successful in allowing patients to die with dignity, this is
done on the backs of nurses:

> If the medical profession has indeed been 'successful' in
> allowing patients to die (whether this has been with or
> without dignity), it is often in the context of ordering
> nurses to perform acts of euthanasia on its behalf. One
> reason why these acts have essentially gone unsecured by
> law enforcement agencies is not so much because of a 'let
> sleeping dogs lie' attitude, but because the medical
> profession has rather cleverly succeeded in upholding an
> almost universal euphemism for prescribing passive and in
> some instances active euthanasia, namely the proverbial
> 'medical order' of 'Nursing Care Only'. This claim
> becomes compelling when it is considered that what
> doctors in fact order is not *nursing care*, but rather the
> *withdrawal* of nursing care'. (p. 266)

According to this it could be argued that, in the case of
Dr Arthur, it was not he who should have been accused
of murder, but the nurse in charge who accepted this
order. Indeed, in the wake of that case, a senior lecturer
in law (Finch, 1981) wrote of nurses that:

> Their position is in truth and in reality enormously difficult.
> There is no defence of mercy killing, and there is equally
> no defence of superior orders. If a nurse commits an act
> which is in fact illegal, whether she intends it to be or
> not, and whatever her motive, she stands to be indicted as
> an accomplice: or perhaps a member of a conspiracy

(agreement) to commit an unlawful act; or even as a principal offender, depending on how far down the road of criminality she has gone. If this sounds frightening that's because it is frightening.

According to the UKCC *Code of Professional Conduct* (1992) 'as a registered nurse, midwife and health visitor, you are personally accountable for your practice and, in the exercise of professional accountability must . . . act always in such a manner as to promote and safeguard the interests and wellbeing of patients and clients'.

It may be that the care given by nurses *only* is indeed the best care, and the appropriate way of treating a particular patient, but this will only be the case after:

- nurses have *themselves* also concluded that this action promotes and safeguards the wellbeing of their patient;
- they have rigorously analysed the morality of their action;
- they have made every effort to establish the patient's preferences.

It is this last point which is again and again the nub, and to which this last part of the chapter is now addressed.

The Caring Relationship

The question of euthanasia is such an important one because it touches people at their most vulnerable point. Many values come and go, but the values which affect life itself are not easily changed nor easily debated. It is easy to be armchair philosophers, but the practice is different. This was clearly evident in a BBC Radio 4 programme in 1991 on 'The Moral Maze'. A panel discussed the subject of euthanasia. and the public was then invited to phone in with their comments. While the studio discussion dealt with the subject in a philosophical way, almost all the people who phoned gave practical examples and viewed the subject from that angle. The difficulty and the sadness was that the two sides were not brought together. Theory and practice were once again divided.

Not only are theory and practice often separate, but so also are logic and emotion, thinking and feeling. Yet if patients are to benefit from any discussion about euthanasia, it is vitally important that all these areas are considered. It was asked earlier, what is humanity — or inhumanity? — and although it may be difficult to answer this question adequately, what is evident is that it is something living, feeling, thinking, capable of choosing and making decisions — in short, experiencing.

So far this chapter has presented the 'thinking' point of view, mostly nourished by other sources and thinkers. To balance this, therefore, it is time to present the 'feeling' view from a more personal point which, although also nourished by others, is less easily quotable because it is perhaps more absorbed and intuited and has been gleaned from various areas.

It is possible to say that ethics has both a feminine and masculine side. By highlighting both it is hoped that they will eventually be seen together in that 'humanity' at the bedside, so to speak, of the person of concern.

It seems that the debate about when life *begins* tends to be for men a question of legality. Does life begin at conception, or at the time when the nervous system has developed sufficiently for the fetus to feel pain, or at some time before or after that? For women the accepted time of when life begins tends to be when they feel the fetus move, that is, when they *experience* life — a particular life — and can relate to it. Thus the relationship to life is a crucial factor.

Can the question of when life *ends* work in the reverse order? Does life end when it legally ends or when the significant relationship with life and in life ends? It tends to be men who invent ever more intricate means of testing, for doubtful cases, when life has ended. This is necessary, but it is only half of what matters. Life does not only end when the law says so. Life may also end for a person when its meaning has ended. This is usually seen when these persons cannot relate meaningfully to other people any more.

In every document, book, article or debate about euthanasia, the point is always made that communication is important, but this communication is more than 'find out what the patient wants'; it is far more than that. A person's wants do not necessarily express that person's needs, and many people express 'wants' in order to please another, and not be seen to be difficult or different.

People express their personalities in their living and in the choices they make about their possibilities. This may all go along very happily for most of the time, until some crisis happens. This may not be a life-threatening crisis; breaking an arm can be just as devastating and insightful for someone. At such moments people need to express themselves. They need to tell their story. Anyone who has fallen ill has a story to tell and needs to tell it. Anyone who is bereaved needs to tell the story of 'how it happened' many times over. This is part of the adjusting; it is therapy. Anyone whose meaning in life has been questioned by illness, disease or loss of any kind needs to talk about it in order to adjust and find a new or different meaning. Some people decide that there is no further meaning, and their 'will to live' atrophies. What people are usually wanting or needing is not quantity of life years, but a meaning in life, and a way of living that meaning.

The debate over a 'right to life' or a 'right to die' is so difficult because we do not 'own' life or death, or a body for that matter; we *are* life; we *are* our bodies. The difficulty is not only one of inadequate words to describe this, but one of inability to express accurately what this means. Questions about euthanasia, therefore, always begin and end with: what is human nature?

Most people find this a too rigorously theoretical question, but when asked what their life means to them they can answer from experience. It means being with a loved person, looking after the children, doing good, helping others, enjoying themselves. When that is not possible any more, for whatever reason, there is a mental, physical and spiritual collapse. Then people who have collapsed may ask for euthanasia, to 'be put out of misery'. The relationship with and to themselves — that is, to life — is so severely damaged that they do not know how to cope and relate to that other, collapsed, side of themselves which they have hardly ever met. 'Ordinary' people may commit suicide at that point. People who are ill and not in a position to take their lives may ask to have it taken for them.

Just as an attempted suicide is so often a cry for help to understand meaning, so it could be said that a call for euthanasia is often also a cry for help. People who are 'collapsed' are not creative. On the contrary, external destruction reflects internal destruction. Yet to know, in the old phrase, that they might soon be 'meeting their Maker' — their creator — while they are uncreative, is very daunting and the only escape seems annihilation, somehow, as if in this way God might not notice.

If there is any answer or any help to be given in this

situation it lies in one area only: listening. It is possible to put this in many different ways: good communication, a caring relationship, dialogue, story-telling, etc.

It does not necessarily take a person skilled in communication to listen, although it could be argued that this would always be an advantage. What matters is that the person who listens also hears what is being said. This means hearing the difference between a cry for help and a statement like 'I'm ready to die' made out of a deep faith.

The main requirement in a listener, be this a nurse, a doctor, a member of the family, or the proverbial cleaner, is that the listener *can* listen totally: one human being listening to another human being; one person being with another person. This demands a great deal, and in this situation most certainly demands that the listener has also faced death and dying. A dying person has above all a right to be heard and listened to, and the obligation or responsibility (response-ability) of the carer is to listen with empathy, and also with the ability to share humanity. What is questioned is the meaning of life; what is answered is out of the meaning of life. What is humanity, or inhumanity, for a person may be heard in that moment.

It is in that listening and hearing that the relationship to and with life is made clear. It is probable that the relationship with the significant other in life is also highlighted. Such listening and hearing is not to be taken lightly; it is at that stage the most delicate, intimate and healing relationship.

Conclusion

By way of a conclusion to the subject of euthanasia a few

statements will be listed here before turning again to the issue of relationship.

The Linacre Centre (1982) is unequivocal in its conclusion: good practice, ie recognising the signs of death, relief of symptoms and team work are paramount. Kennedy (1990), an ardent enthusiast for voluntary euthanasia, would like to see supplies of living wills in every doctor's surgery, and that patients should complete and return them (p. 47). Johnstone (1989), writing from a nursing perspective and addressing nurses, believes that:

> we need to be much more honest about the nature of death-inducing acts being performed in our hospitals, and be considerably more careful about the grounds upon which and ways in which these are performed. It is not acceptable that euthanasia is disguised under the euphemism 'nursing care only'. (p. 271)

She also urges 'society' to be clear about whether euthanasia is permissible and under what conditions. The fact that society has tacitly conceded to it already is not enough to make it also morally permissible.

It is widely believed that euthanasia is practised legally in Holland. This is not strictly true. What happens is that the Dutch Supreme Court has laid down guidelines for doctors. If these are followed, the acts of euthanasia will most likely not be prosecuted (*Bulletin of Medical Ethics*, 53, p. 8).

At present (November 1991), the European Parliament is discussing a 'Motion for a resolution on care of the terminally ill', brought by a Dutch member. This resolution, reproduced in full here, may go some way to making the law on euthanasia clearer.

Motion for a resolution on care of the terminally ill.

(Reprinted with permission of the Editor, *Bulletin of Medical Ethics*.)

The European Parliament

— having regard to the motion for a resolution by Mrs Van Hemeldonck on counselling for the terminally ill,

— having regard to its resolution of 19 January 1984 on a European Charter on the Rights of Patients,

— having regard to its resolution of 13 May 1986 on a European Charter for Children in Hospital,

— having regard to the report of the Committee on the Environment, Public Health and Consumer Protection,

A. whereas human life is founded on *dignity and spirituality*, and cannot therefore be reduced to merely *natural* functions, ie the functions of vegetative existence,

B. whereas the death of an individual is determined by the cessation of cerebral function, even where biological functions continue,

C. whereas cerebral function determines the *level of consciousness* which in turn defines a human being,

D. whereas attempts to cure at all costs, even though an illness is incurable at the present stage of medical knowledge, must be avoided, as must inexorable treatment, which offends against the dignity of the individual,

E. whereas it is proposed that the European Charter on the Rights of Patients should enshrine 'the right to a dignified death',

F. whereas it is proposed that the European Charter for Children in Hospital should include 'the right to be protected from unnecessary medical treatment and physical or emotional distress',

G. whereas physical pain is useless and destructive, and may offend against human dignity,

H. whereas every means available should be used to

combat pain, in particular the use of appropriate drugs such as morphine and its derivatives, administered according to the rules in force,

I. whereas a lonely death in hospital has now sadly become a frequent occurrence,

J. whereas it is essential for all forms of palliative care to be provided to patients once a cure has become impossible and specific medical treatment is no longer effective,

K. whereas the provision of palliative care is not the responsibility of the medical institution alone but also of family, friends . . . and society in general,

L. whereas the desire for eternal sleep is not a negation of life but a request for an end to an existence which illness has finally robbed of all dignity,

1. Considers that, in the interests of sound medical practice, it is necessary for medical staff, doctors, nurses and nursing auxiliaries to be trained so as to enable them to:

(a) treat and cure patients suffering from curable acute conditions;

(b) treat and give the best possible support to patients suffering from chronic conditions;

(c) provide appropriate care for incurable patients whose illness has become refractory to any specific treatment;

(d) have an understanding and caring attitude towards patients nearing death;

2. To this end, call on the Commission to encourage exchanges both of experiences and of staff under existing programmes with a view to widening knowledge of palliative care and improving techniques;

3. Calls for the rapid establishment in every hospital service in the European Community of palliative care units, and the subsequent establishment of rooms for palliative or continuing care in all departments dealing with the seriously ill;

4. Calls upon the Commission to carry out a study of hospitals in the European Community with particular reference to this type of care;

5. Calls for account to be taken, in allocating hospital building aid from the European Regional Development Fund, of the creation of palliative care rooms and subsequently units and of the existence of structures to enable seriously ill patients to be with their family and/or those they love until the end of their lives;

6. Calls for all possible steps to be taken to promote treatment at home whenever medically possible;

7. Calls for encouragement and aid to be given to voluntary associations like those in Italy, the United Kingdom and Belgium which effectively support the medical profession by helping to care for patients in the terminal stages of their lives;

8. Considers that, in the absence of any curative treatment and following the failure of palliative care correctly provided at both psychological and medical level, each time a fully conscious patient insistently and repeatedly requests an end to an existence which has for him been robbed of all dignity and each time a team of doctors created for that purpose establishes the impossibility of providing further specific care, the request should be satisfied without thereby involving any breach of respect for human life;

9. Calls on the European Community to initiate a wideranging round-table discussion among those with ethical, political and medical authority on the respect due to the patient at the end of his life;

10. Instructs its President to forward this resolution to the Commission and Council.

Explanatory statement

In spite of remarkable progress in medicine over the last forty years, some diseases remain incurable. Care of the terminally ill, an area long neglected, should be considered as one of the objectives of modern high-technology medicine, which must not forget that it is exclusively concerned with people, whose lives are defined by dignity.

Any debate on care of the terminally ill should be based on the following premises:
— The life of a human being cannot be reduced to its merely natural functions: the beating of the heart, the circulation of the blood, the breathing of the lungs . . . it is the functioning of the brain which determines the level of consciousness, and it is in turn the level of consciousness which defines human existence. The cessation of cerebral function means the death of the individual, even when his biological functions continue.
— The desire to cure at all costs even when an illness is incurable at the current stage of medical knowledge must be avoided, as must inexorable treatment, a medical failing related to intellectual stubbornness which has led in some cases to unreasonable suffering being inflicted in the name of political expediency.
— Pain is useless and destructive, and can in most cases be overcome by the administration of appropriate drugs. There is no reason to be afraid of using powerful pain-killers, principally morphine and its derivatives.

Among the medical profession, care of the terminally ill hides behind the term 'palliative care': such care should be opted for when a cure has become impossible because specific treatment has become ineffective. Palliative care consists in reducing the symptoms of the disease without acting on its cause. It makes it possible to fight against pain, discomfort and fear.

Experimental palliative care units have been set up, first in Britain, and later in Canada, the USA and France. These units should play a pilot role, instead of being rare exceptions. Each hospital department should include a few palliative care rooms for patients of this kind, who should not be grouped together in specialised, ghetto-like wards . . .

It is undeniable that in the interests of sound medical practice and proper palliative (or continuing) care, all medical staff must be trained to enable them to:
— treat and cure patients suffering from acute curable conditions;
— treat and give the best possible support to patients suffering from chronic conditions;
— provide appropriate care for incurable patients who are no longer responding to any specific treatment;
— have an understanding and caring attitude towards patients approaching death.

The provision of palliative care for the terminally ill is not the responsibility of the medical institution alone but also of family, friends, and acquaintances and society in general. In Italy and the United Kingdom, voluntary associations (Vidas and the Hospice movement) have developed aid structures for the seriously ill: regular hospital visits, premises to receive patients who have been permitted to leave hospital, etc. Such initiatives should be encouraged and developed throughout the Community.

Now that a lonely death in hospital has sadly become all too frequent, everything ought to be done to encourage caring for the terminally ill at home. It is highly desirable that hospitals in the EEC should set up reception structures to enable the seriously ill to be with their family and those they love until they die.

It is dignity which defines a human life. When, at the end of a long illness against which he has fought courageously, the patient asks the doctor to terminate an existence which has lost all dignity for him, and the doctor decides in all conscience to assist him and to ease the final hours of his life by allowing him to fall asleep peacefully and finally, this medical and humane assistance (sometimes called euthanasia) is respect for human life.

Bulletin of Medical Ethics (1991) no. 69, pp. 25–7.

To legislate for euthanasia is an almost impossible task. Proposals have been made whereby a patient would submit an application, accompanied by two medical certificates, a special referee would interview the patient, and if the referee were satisfied, the patient could be issued with a certificate, and then be killed seven days later in the presence of an official witness (Rachels 1986, p. 183). Clearly, this is far too complicated.

Rachels suggests that legalising euthanasia could be done 'the other way round', so to speak, by making:

a plea of mercy-killing acceptable as a defence against a charge of homicide in much the same way that a plea of self-defence is acceptable. . . . someone charged with homicide . . . could plead mercy-killing; and then, if it could be shown that the victim while competent requested death, and that the victim was suffering from a painful terminal illness, the defendant would also be acquitted. (p. 185)

Under this proposal, 'the need to write complicated legislation permitting euthanasia is bypassed' (p. 187).

In the field of morality it is always easier to say what should *not* be done than what *should* be done. It is easy enough to say 'do not murder'; it is much less easy to say, and do: listen to the person, hear what is being said, respect the person.

Good practice is necessarily what everyone wants and should have. Codes of Practice go some way to laying down the basics, but eventually it is the individual carer who is in a relationship and situation with another person, and it is that which counts.

Life is the most precious thing we have and are, and it is so precious because it is so transient. The quest for the meaning of life is a person's ultimate quest. The handicapped, malformed and 'incompetent' challenge that meaning in particular, and therefore the question of euthanasia for these people is a thorny issue.

Listening to someone who has asked for euthanasia is therefore also the most complex and challenging task. To hear someone tell of their meaning or search for it, or to help that person to find it, is not something done 'cold' by someone who simply 'has' life; it is done by someone who is *living*. Ultimately, a person should not be asking for the meaning *of* his or her life, but must recognise that it is he or she who is being questioned. A person is questioned by life, and that person can only answer to life by *answering* for his or her own life (Frankl 1962, p. 111). To witness this is awesome.

Although the discussion has focused on *life*, something similar is true also of death. Death challenges us, not as something from outside, but as something which *is* us. Thiroux (1977) sums up the value of life principle by saying 'Human beings should revere life and accept death' (p. 124). How we do that indeed characterises us as individuals and as a society.

References

Age Concern (1988) *The Living Will: Consent to treatment at the end of life*. London, Edward Arnold.

Andrews, J. (1989) Whose right is it, anyway? *Nursing Times,* **85**(47): 24.

Beauchamp, T.L. and Davidson, A.I. (1979). The definition of euthanasia. *The Journal of Medicine and Philosophy,* **4**(3): 294–312.

Bulletin of Medical Ethics
38, May 1988: 13.
53, Sept/Oct 1989: 8.
60, August 1990: 23.
61, September 1990: 19.
62, October 1990: 20.
63, November 1990: 6.
65, February 1991: 3, 4/6.
69, June 1991: 6.
70, August 1991: 8.

Campbell, R. and Collinson, D. (1988) *Ending Lives*. Oxford, Blackwell Ltd.

Camus, A. (1955) *The Myth of Sisyphus*. London, Hamish Hamilton.

Daily Telegraph (1991) 31 August.

Duncan, A.S., Dunstan, G.R. and Welbourn, R.B. (1977) *Dictionary of Medical Ethics*. London, Darton, Longman & Todd.

Finch, J. (1981) The Arthur Case. In Darbyshire, P. (1986) Angels of mercy?, *Nursing Times,* **82**(8): 49–52.

Fletcher, J. (1977) In Downing, A. B. (ed.), *Euthanasia and the Right to Die*, (pp. 65–6), London, Peter Owen.

Frankl, V. (1962) *Man's Search for Meaning*. London, Hodder and Stoughton.

Johnstone, M-J. (1989) *Bioethics, a Nursing Perspective*. Sydney, W.B. Saunders.

Kennedy, L. (1990) *Euthanasia*. London, Chatto and Windus.

Linacre Centre (1982) *Euthanasia and Clinical Practice*. Report of a Working Party. London, The Linacre Centre.

Lockwood, M. (1985) Who is to live? *New Society*, **71**(1151): 94.

Mahoney, J. (1984) *Bioethics and Belief.* London, Sheed and Ward.

Miller, P.J. (1987) Death with dignity and the right to die: sometimes doctors have a duty to hasten death. *Journal of Medical Ethics*, **13**(2): 81–5.

Rachels, J. (1986) *The End of Life.* Oxford, Oxford University Press.

Thiroux, J. (1977) *Ethics, Theory and Practice.* Encino CA, Glencoe Publishing Co.

UKCC (1992) *Code of Professional Conduct* (3rd edn.). London, UKCC.

US President's Commission Report (1983) *Deciding to Forego Life-sustaining Treatment.* Washington DC, US Government Printing Office.

Further Reading

Age Concern (1988) *The Living Will: Consent to treatment at the end of life.* London, Edward Arnold.

A useful book setting out the pros, cons and practicalities of euthanasia.

Campbell, R. and Collinson, D. (1988) *Ending Lives.* Oxford, Blackwell Ltd.

One of the Open University books for the course *Life and Death*, this is a philosophical treatise about suicide and euthanasia.

Johnstone, M-J. (1989) *Bioethics, a Nursing Perspective.* Sydney, W.B. Saunders.

A clear and well–argued book by a nurse on all aspects of ethics. Chapter 8 deals particularly with abortion and euthanasia.

Kennedy, L. (1990) *Euthanasia*. London, Chatto and Windus.

One of the 'Counter-Blast' series of book, this volume is very readable and entirely *for* voluntary euthanasia.

Linacre Centre (1982) *Euthanasia and Clinical Practice*. Report of a Working Party. London, The Linacre Centre.

This Report, written some time ago, and entirely from a Roman Catholic standpoint, is a very useful addition to the subject of euthanasia.

Mahoney, J. (1984) *Bioethics and Belief*. London, Sheed and Ward.

Chapter 2 of this excellent book by a Roman Catholic theologian is about death and dying, and is closely argued and often pithy in character.

Rachels, J. (1986) *The End of Life*. Oxford, Oxford University Press.

This book is recommended as 'interesting, informed, and readable'. It is all that, and also often controversial, making it stimulating and challenging.

Thiroux, J. (1977) *Ethics, Theory and Practice*. Encino CA, Glencoe Publishing Co.

A useful text on all aspects of ethics. Chapter 8 deals with death. Each chapter contains cases for study and discussion and exercises for review.

Useful Addresses

The Voluntary Euthanasia Society
13 Prince of Wales Terrace
London W8 5PG
Telephone: 071–937 7770

Natural Death Centre
20 Hebar Road
Cricklewood
London NW2 6AA

A non-profit-making association aiming to improve the quality of
dying. The Centre eventually wants to formulate a 'declaration of
the dying person's rights'.

Index

Index